Healthy Schools,
Healthy Futures

Information on how to obtain copies of this book is available at
www.thompsonbooks.com
Phone: 416.766.2763
Fax: 416.766.0398

Publisher: Keith Thompson
Managing Editor: Jane McNulty
Editor: Paul McNulty

Jane and Paul McNulty wish to dedicate their work on this book not only to the spirit and memory of Dr. Andy Anderson, but also to the spirit and memory of their mother **Marie (McNamara) McNulty** *(1925–2017), who devoted 37 years of her life to enhancing the health and well-being of the Grade One students entrusted to her care in Saint John, New Brunswick.*

Library and Archives Canada Cataloguing in Publication

Anderson, Andy Thomas, author

Healthy schools, healthy futures : make your school a health-promoting community / Andy Anderson, Associate Professor, Elementary (Physical and Health Education), O.I.S.E., University of Toronto [1996–2007], James Mandigo, Vice Provost and Professor, Faculty of Applied Health Sciences, Brock University, Doug Gleddie, Associate Professor, Faculty of Education, University of Alberta.

Includes bibliographical references and index.
ISBN 978-1-55077-191-6 (softcover)

1. School children—Health and hygiene. 2. Health education. 3. Health promotion. I. Mandigo, James, author II. Gleddie, Doug, 1971–, author III. Title.

LB3405.A53 2018 371.7'1 C2018-904058-0

We acknowledge the support of the Government of Canada through the Canada Book Fund for our publishing activities. We also acknowledge the support of the Government of Ontario through the Ontario Media Development Corporation.

Canadä

Printed in Canada.

1 2 3 4 5 23 22 21 20 19 18

Healthy Schools, Healthy Futures

Make Your School a Health-Promoting Community

Andy Anderson

Associate Professor, Elementary (Physical and Health Education),
O.I.S.E., University of Toronto [1996–2007]

James Mandigo

Vice Provost and Professor, Faculty of Applied Health Sciences,
Brock University

Doug Gleddie

Associate Professor, Faculty of Education,
University of Alberta

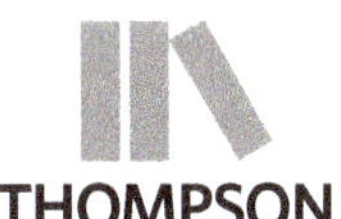

THOMPSON

Table of Contents

About the Authors

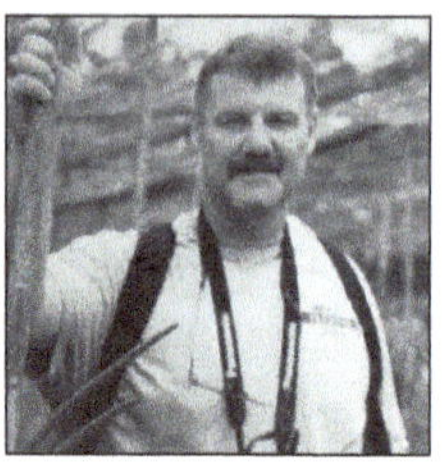

Andy Anderson
Associate Professor, Elementary (Physical and Health Education), O.I.S.E., University of Toronto [1996–2007]

Andy Anderson was a distinguished author and scholar in the health and physical education field. He published extensively in the area of health-promoting schools and made presentations to teachers and academics around the world. Andy passed away from brain cancer in August, 2007.

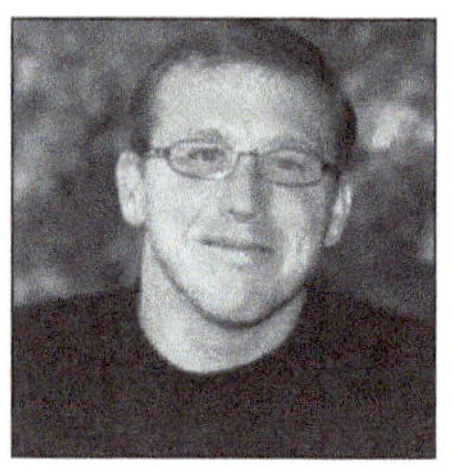

James Mandigo
Vice Provost and Professor, Department of Kinesiology, Faculty of Applied Health Sciences, Brock University

James Mandigo's research focuses on youth and the development of life skills through physical education and sport. He is a past president of Ophea and has earned numerous awards, including an Award for Distinguished Teaching and an Award for Teaching Excellence.

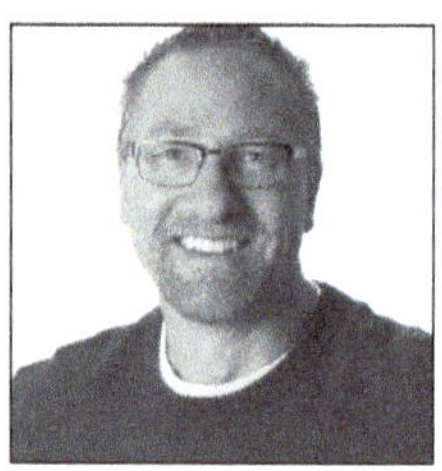

Doug Gleddie
Associate Professor, Department of Elementary Education, Faculty of Education, University of Alberta

Doug Gleddie's research includes physical literacy, teacher education, and narratives of movement and physical education. He is a past director of Ever Active Schools and a recent winner of the Provost's Award for Undergraduate Teaching Excellence.

Acknowledgements

Dr. Finney Cherian, University of Windsor
Dr. John Corlett, MacEwan University
Christa Costas-Bradstreet, CCB Consulting, Burlington
Dr. Nancy Francis, Brock University
Ashley Johnson, Queen's University
Kim Sanderson, Edmonton Parks and Recreation
Carol Scaini, Treeline Public School
Marg Schwartz, APPLE Schools
Dr. Joanna Sheppard, University of the Fraser Valley
June Sowden, Six Nations Reserve
Dr. Amanda Stanec, Move Live Learn
Ontario Physical and Health Education Association (Ophea)
Physical and Health Education Canada (PHE Canada)

Andy's Scholarly Impact

"Every child is a champion." This was the motto for Andy's work around the world. Whether it was teaching pre-service students at the Ontario Institute for Studies in Education, conducting workshops with teachers in the Caribbean or Latin America, or playing with children from a local orphanage in Thailand, Andy truly believed that every child has talents, dreams, and hopes which, if channelled in the right direction, can make a difference in that child's life and the lives of others.

Andy was a leader in health and physical education around the world. As an associate professor at the University of Toronto and an adjunct professor at Brock University, Andy made a significant and profound impact upon his profession. In May, 2007, Andy was awarded the prestigious North American Scholars Award, which recognizes outstanding professionals within the allied professions of health education, physical education, recreation, sport, and dance in North America. Andy also received several teaching awards at the University of Toronto and the 2005 R.Tait McKenzie Award of Honour, Physical and Health Education Canada's most prestigious award. In 2008, Physical and Health Education Canada renamed their young professional award to the Dr. Andy Anderson Young Professional Award in recognition of Andy's dedication to inspiring future leaders. The award is "... presented to one professional per provincial association that best epitomizes exemplary work on behalf of the physical and health education profession."

Andy's achievements extended far beyond the borders of our country; he shared his scholarship at international conferences and workshops in Australia, the Caribbean, Mexico, El Salvador, Finland, Puerto Rico, Thailand, and the United States.

The legacy of Andy's work has and will continue to have a profound influence on his profession around the world for generations to come. This book represents a combination of Andy's final words as a scholar and the legacy of his work—he passed away from brain cancer in August, 2007. Although he was not able to finish this book, much of the material was written by Andy. The current examples provided through various vignettes demonstrate how his work has continued to shape the thinking and activiites of students, educators, families, and communities around the world.

> **Andy was the consummate educator and we hope that you continue to be inspired by Andy's vision for our schools to be a place where children and youth can learn the skills to care for themselves and to care for others.**
>
> — James Mandigo
> *Vice Provost and Professor, Brock University*

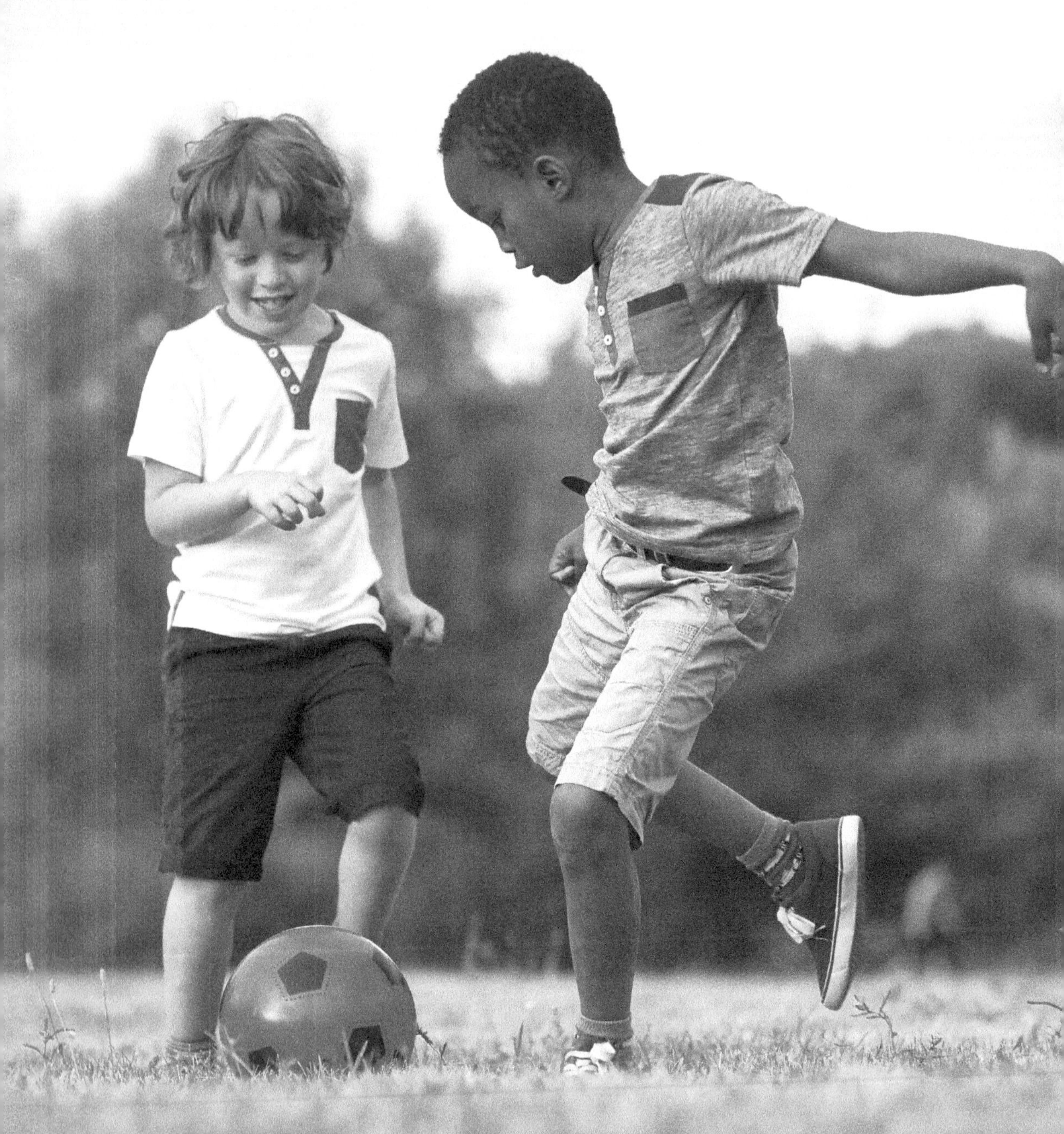

1

Health Education in Our Schools

Shaping our children's lives and futures

What makes someone healthy? Is it simply the absence of disease? Or is good health rooted in the quality of life an individual leads—not only from a physical perspective, but also from social, cognitive, and spiritual perspectives?

Civil rights leader Dr. Martin Luther King Jr. is remembered as one of the most influential activists for social change in our time. In the face of civil unrest and at the expense of his own personal safety, Dr. King pursued a dream to ensure that all people had the opportunity to lead lives that were not only free, but that were enriched. Imagine a society in which everyone has access to the nutrition they need. Imagine a society in which everyone has access to high-quality education. Imagine a society that celebrates and embraces not only its own culture, but the cultures of all people. Imagine a society in which everyone enjoys equality and freedom and is treated with dignity and respect. Such a society would truly be the healthiest place on Earth.

Take this dream a step further and imagine a community in which the school is at the centre of nurturing and fostering the health of all its members. Imagine a school in which students, staff, parents, guardians, and all who regularly interact within the school learn not only how to care for their own health, but also how to look out for the health of others and the environments in which they live. This vision of health and the role that schools can play within each of our communities is at the heart of this book.

The United Nations was formed in 1945 in the aftermath of World War II as an organization to bring nations together to discuss their differences through diplomatic and peaceful means rather than resorting to the violence of war. Embedded in the 111 articles of the UN Charter is the central importance of health. This recognition of the significance of health led the UN to create the World Health Organization (WHO) in 1948 as its principal public-health arm. WHO's first director-general was Dr. Brock Chisholm, a Canadian psychiatrist and former federal deputy minister of health.

The World Health Organization (WHO) defines health as "a state of complete physical, mental and social well-being and not merely the absence of disease or infirmity."

With the world still recovering from the devastating effects of World War II, WHO needed a definition of health that was not just about the absence of disease, but also about striving toward overall positive well-being. In 1948, millions of people were still struggling to cope with physical bodily injury caused by the violence of war, with mental horrors inflicted on them during the conflict, and with social challenges rebuilding towns, cities, and countries in the absence of family, friends, and loved ones who were killed. Amidst these conditions, WHO recognized the importance of a holistic view of human health. Just as the creation of the United Nations was intended to prevent another world war, the creation of WHO was intended to focus efforts on how nations can work together on "the preventative side of health … not merely on the absence of illness" (Sze, 1998, 29–34).

Its modern definition influenced by WHO, health is now seen as a concept that extends well beyond disease prevention and eradication. Current perspectives on health promotion in Canada and around the world have been strongly influenced by the Ottawa Charter for Health Promotion (WHO, 1986). The charter asserts in part:

> Defined as a resource for living, health is not something a person waits for passively. Rather, it is an ongoing part of our lives, something we actively assert, strive for, and convey throughout our lives. The word *resource* means to revitalize; hence the notion of health is a way to enhance our lives. Too often risk avoidance, harm reduction campaigns make "risk" the centre of attention. In contrast, health promotion efforts prefer to focus on enabling factors or the reward that comes from putting people's talents, imaginations, and hopes into action so they can assume greater control over the conditions that enable them to lead a healthy life.

This chapter introduces health within the context of schools and the role that education can play to help empower individuals to make healthy choices not only for themselves, but with consideration for others and the environments in which we live. If we have any hope of creating a healthy society such as the one that WHO envisions, schools must play a central role within our communities. Schools have the potential not only to equip the next generation of children and youth with the requisite skills to make healthy choices, but also to serve as a hub within a community that supports its own healthy development.

School-based health promotion is a process whereby teachers, students, staff, parents, guardians, and community partners work together to develop programs, resources, and activities that address health issues in a manner that is (a) comprehensive (e.g., by integrating changes in individual behaviours, skills, knowledge, and attitudes with modifications to the environment) and (b) consistent with education- related and school-related goals and mandates.

When included in the professional practice of educators, health promotion as a conceptual model provides a lens through which to explore and guide academic study, school culture, community partnerships, innovative design, and improvement strategies, along with the coordination of supports and services. As such, health promotion inspires and activates intellectual, social, and communal growth.

Effective health promotion is more than preparing young people to reduce the risk of preventable injury, illness, and disease. It should also encourage people to be fully engaged in knowledge- and community-building efforts that feed into the development of aptitudes, attitudes, and conditions that result in healthy living. In other words, health promotion is ideally an opportunity for growth and progress in many areas rather than a program of treatment modalities.

Throughout the world the cost of providing health care is enormous. In 2016, the Canadian Institute for Health Information estimated that total health-care expenditures reached $228 billion, 11% of Canada's total GDP (Canadian Institute for Health Information, 2016). Canada ranks fifth in the world behind the United States, France, Germany, and Sweden in health-care spending as a percentage of GDP. Health-care costs in Ontario alone represent 46% of the provincial budget and are expected to reach 80% by 2030 without a significant intervention (Drummond, 2013).

Attention to the cost of health care, both in terms of the impact on an individual's quality of life and the impact on a society's economy and social capital, is critical. Here, it is important to keep in mind the essential role that teachers play. Teachers teach. They provide experiences that enable students to learn. Great teachers are one of the most important determinants of a great school, engaging and meaningful student learning, and young people's overall success in life. Teacher excellence is therefore a significant part of nation building and efforts, both globally and locally, to address a multiplicity of health issues.

The Dimensions of Health

When people speak about health, the subject is often categorized into four dimensions: physical, social, mental, and spiritual. These dimensions present a way to orient, organize, and act to improve learning in schools. To construct a more complete understanding of what happens at your school, consider not only how each dimension is evident in the classroom or school, but also how each dimension interacts with the others.

- **Physical health** refers to the condition of human biological systems—skeletal, muscular, nervous, respiratory, cardiovascular, lymphatic, digestive, endocrine, urinary, integumentary, and reproductive. In schools, students learn about the role of each body system and ways in which they can support the healthy functioning of these systems. For example, students can make connections to how physical activities in which they participate both during and after school can have a positive influence on their skeletal, muscular, and cardiovascular health. As another example, students can learn about the importance of making healthy choices for themselves and others to prevent sexually transmitted infections and to protect their reproductive health.

- Social health in schools refers to the relationships that students and teachers enjoy in class, in hallways and lunchrooms, and during school activities. Social health refers as well to feelings of belonging, caring about, and being cared for by others. In one school, students shaved their heads as a show of support for a fellow student who had lost his hair following cancer treatment—this is a powerful example of social health in action.
- Mental health is defined by the Centre for Addiction and Mental Health (CAMH) as the "ability to enjoy life and deal with the challenges you face everyday—whether that involves making choices and decisions, adapting to and coping in difficult situations, or talking about your needs and desires" (Ballon, 2003, 11). In schools, mental health refers to helping students acquire coping and self-management skills that will foster resilience, while at the same time develop the recognition skills needed to identify signs of mental illness and where and how to seek help. Bandura (1997) argues that self-efficacy is not just the skills we acquire but rather our judgments as to what we can do with those skills. In other words, with the support of their teachers, students can learn to cope with pressures to meet standards, pass tests, and live up to personal and parental expectations. This kind of self-efficacy can strengthen the confidence that students and teachers have in their ability to face these challenges as an integral part of the student achievement process.
- Spiritual health refers to the overall culture and character of a school. The importance of spirituality is symbolized in the medicine wheel that is central to the worldviews of Indigenous peoples. The medicine wheel describes spirituality as the "stewardship of the Earth and recognition that all of life (and the universe) is interrelated" (Toulouse, 2016, 10). Through the lens of spiritual health, teachers can explore key questions such as: What set of values (or higher ground) does this school represent in students' lives? What place does this school occupy in the community? What does this school hold in esteem regarding the contributions of students and teachers to both education and society? What does the school feel about its work: pride? frustration? disappointment? enthusiasm? Do students feel a sense of hope? How are dreams and achievements celebrated? As a result of their learning experiences, do students feel a sense of wonder? Are they curious about how new knowledge speaks to them and their lives? Are they better able to receive the key messages and enter into a dialogue with the various authors and texts presented to them in their various areas of study?

Together, the dimensions of health can be used as templates to plan, review, and create new ways to teach, as well as manage and assess what is happening in schools. According to the foregoing dimensions, a healthy learner is someone who:

- has faith in their own capabilities as a learner
- values learning
- enjoys coming to school
- is ready to learn—is rested, is nourished, and feels safe
- accepts challenges
- uses a variety of learning and study strategies to take control of their learning

Care for Self, Others, and the Environment

> ***The challenge to humanity is to adopt new ways of thinking, new ways of acting, new ways of organizing itself in society—in short, new ways of living.*** —*Our Creative Diversity* (Perez et al., 1997)

In her book *Harvest of Hope* (2006), Jane Goodall tells a story about visiting a First Nations community during a special event that involves a ritual of giving and sacrifice. A major part of Nevada Washo life is centred around something called "Giveaway"—the way of all life. This community's belief is that two-legged, four-legged, the birds of the air, the fish of the sea, all know that to be centred they must participate in the Giveaway. Everything in the universe practises Giveaway in one way or another. Members of this community believe that "without sacrifice there is no real expression of love." "We give away to friends, relatives, and even to people we may have never met before. We give away for many reasons. We give away if we feel good, or are thankful, or if someone is in need. We express thanks, or attempt to spread the good feelings we have, by giving gifts.

> Part of the ceremonial activities involves the killing of a buffalo from the herd that has assembled in the valley below the camp. After much dancing and singing, a group of hunters prepared their spears and prayer stick and move solemnly toward the herd. The singing stops as the valley falls deadly quiet. The medicine man raised the prayer stick and asked the buffalo from the herd, whose turn it was to give away, to come forward. A large young bull began to walk toward him. As he prayed, the bull walked slowly past the elders and headed straight for the medicine man. The medicine man handed the prayer stick to one of the elders and placed his right hand out to accept the buffalo's sacrifice. When a buffalo comes to offer the Giveaway, he will place his head in the hand of the medicine man and then drop his head to die. But just before the young bull reached his hand an older, larger bull came from out of the middle of the herd, and running in front of the young bull he pushed him away and placed his head in the medicine man's hand. Some of the herd came and circled the young bull as though to hold him back. It was quite an amazing sight. There is no greater love than this—that a man (in this case an animal) lay down his life for his friends. (Goodall, 2008)

The story of the Giveaway Buffalo introduces the notion of health mindedness as part of how we, as humans, can also prepare ourselves for care and service beyond self. A perspective of care shifts attention away from a disease orientation and biomedical outlooks on health to an emphasis on empathy and compassion. Consider, for example, how a unit on healthy eating might be designed when the expectation is that students will have greater knowledge about, and concern for, the relationship between food production and energy consumption. Are agricultural and food marketing practices that are designed to manufacture massive amounts of processed food products, overpackaging, and larger sizes doing more harm than good? Exactly how much does it cost—both economically and environmentally—to make strawberries available to consumers in Canada in January?

Health mindedness, therefore, is an orientation to thinking about the world with care for self, others, and the environment as a critical focus. With care for self and others in mind, students are encouraged to adopt patterns and orientations in their thinking that:

- invite students to be mindful of their behaviours and habits of consumption, including and beyond personal use
- enable them to think critically and alternatively about their health options
- challenge them to (re)examine the origins of their beliefs about health outcomes in relation to an ethic of care
- prepare students to relate their knowledge and skills to the practice of health promotion

A health-minded motorist drives with care for self, environment, and others in mind. A health-minded educator develops learning experiences that deepen and broaden students' understanding of the relationship between subject-matter knowledge and care for self and others. Health mindedness broadens and deepens the relevance and meaningfulness of what is taught. Accordingly, health-minded educators ask themselves: "How will I teach this unit in such a way that students think differently about themselves—respect themselves, feel confident about their choices and efforts to succeed, see the presence of this knowledge in their day-to-day lives, and understand how this knowledge affects them?"

Health Mindedness and Intellectual Character

Health mindedness contributes to the development of what Ritchhart (2002) refers to as intellectual character. Skills associated with intellectual character include the dispositions and habits of mind associated with lifelong learning, problem solving, and decision making. He writes: "In contrast to viewing intelligence as a set of capacities or even skills, the concept of intellectual character recognizes the role of attitude and affect in our everyday cognition and the importance of developed patterns of behaviour." (Ritchhart, 18). Ritchhart writes further about intellectual character as:

- Virtues and passions. fair-mindedness, fervour for getting to the bottom of things, sympathetic listening, drive to seek out evidence, intellectual sense of justice

- **Habits of creative, self-regulated, and critical thinking.** engagement in tasks even when the answers or solutions are not apparent, generating new ways of viewing a situation outside the boundaries of standard conventions, sensitivity to others' feelings and level of knowledge
- **Key dispositions.** persistence, empathic listening, finding humour, and taking the total situation into account

Like "intelligent behaviour" that Dewey (1995) discusses, intellectual character moves learning beyond the narrow accumulation of discrete facts toward engagement in the development of skills and thought patterns needed to make discriminating and careful choices. Intellectual character can be described in terms of three areas of development:

- **Creative thinking.** looking out, up, around, and about (open-mindedness and curiosity)
- **Reflective thinking.** looking within (metacognition)
- **Critical thinking.** looking at, through, and in between (search for truth and understanding, strategic and skeptical attitude)

These ways of thinking enable students to be smarter (detect bias), stronger (make decisions in relation to goals and values, not persuasion), and safer (assert their own and others' rights and entitlements). What might be taken for granted or at face value now comes under scrutiny. Propositions and claims now undergo tough questioning: Whose interests are being served? What are the hidden messages? Why am I interested in this decision?

Health mindedness invites thinking on several planes: philosophical, political, social, and moral. Consider, for example, the outcomes of a student-led initiative to change the menu in a school's cafeteria to promote healthy eating. As active citizens advocating for health, students learn the importance of well-designed change projects and the need for commitment by all stakeholders: parents, guardians, students, support staff, and teachers. Students must also decide whether to seek partnerships with external entities that may be needed to achieve their goals—community health agencies and food-service distributors, for example. Students engaged in a study of the change process are often startled to learn that the best ideas are not always the ones that are the most successful, that small changes are important, and that behavioural change precedes changes in beliefs and attitudes.

Four frogs sat on a log. One decided to jump off. How many frogs are left? Four! Deciding to do something and actually doing something are not the same. Learning about health should involve closing the gap between knowing and doing—and valuing.

Well-Being and Being Well

Perspective matters. How we view the world determines the tools we use to build knowledge, develop reasoning skills, and respond to change. With health in mind, we can "qualify" our thinking. Under these conditions, health becomes a way of reasoning and making judgments about how we choose to live our lives. What we do for the sake of health tells us about the kind of knowledge we prefer to work with. Consider the difference between cure for health and care for health. In education, care for health links learning to making decisions about how we want to live our lives. Health practices tell us about a person's background (such as culture and ethnicity), upbringing (e.g., family experiences), and outlook (such as ambitions, hopes, and sense of purpose in life).

> ***There is nothing in a caterpillar that tells you it's going to be a butterfly.***—Buckminster Fuller

Centuries ago, Aristotle proposed the notion that the good person lives well. Living well, according to Aristotle, is determined by the relationships we enjoy within our family, community, and society. The goods needed to live well fall into three categories: goods of the body, goods of the soul, and external goods. Goods of the body include such things as health, fitness, strength, and suppleness. Examples of goods of the soul include virtues, intelligence, and wit. External goods include wealth, property, civil status, and training. Combined, these goods represent what it means for a citizen to live well (Glouberman, 2001).

Aristotle recognized not only a hierarchy of goodness but also a relationship between particular goods and virtues. According to Aristotle, virtues are modes of choice, ways of bringing ends into action. They are dispositions of the individual, and require various goods as part of their capacity. Fitness and strength, for example, are goods of the body that enable the virtue of courage. A weak or unhealthy person will have less capacity to act courageously. Similarly, intelligence is a means to the end of a virtue such as courage. Education in the science of politics is an external good to the end of engagement in government (Glouberman, 2001). In the context of health education, preparing students to think critically about health issues enables them to find their voice, take a stand, and speak out for change. The virtues that students display in this process stand in relation to the ultimate end of eudaimonia, that is, well-being, living the good life, being a virtuous person, excellence, or happiness (Glouberman, 2001).

For Aristotle, well-being is not a state, but an activity. Living a good life involves action and engagement in one's society. Living well, therefore, is bound up in the interaction between individuals and their social context. How well people interpret and respond to their environments marks the health of both the individual and their society. Accordingly, education for health must involve the acquisition of certain goods (skills and dispositions) that enable a person to figure out how to respond to what is or is not happening between people, circumstances, and resources. Put simply, education for health is about learning how to progress toward aspirations, a preferred future, and self-actualization.

SUCCESS STORY

Teaching with Health in Mind: Crossing the Volcano

By John Corlett

Consider the following game called Crossing the Volcano. We often played this game in El Salvador to help children and youth there make connections to health issues such as respect for others, which is at the heart of reducing interpersonal violence.

To play, teams of four to eight students begin at a starting point within an open space and a target location that they all must reach. The space between—20 metres or more—is the volcano and they must cross it together. They are given readily available, low- or no-cost implements (such as hoops, water bottles, bean bags, newspapers, skipping ropes) from which to build an ever-unfolding bridge. Upon leaving the starting point, each person, while moving across the volcano, must be supported by one of the implements at all times. Students must work together, moving in a line, one after the other, balancing, holding on to one another, and ensuring that no one slips from the implements to meet their demise in the volcano. The group will typically reach the other side relatively easily, each member crossing safely with the help of teammates and their supporting implements.

Then all the students must cross back over the volcano, but this time with one or two fewer implements than they had the first time. This is more challenging, requiring more planning before each step is taken and requiring individuals to take more risks on behalf of others in the group. The process continues: the group size remains the same as does the challenge, while the resources to solve the problem of helping everyone to arrive successfully on the other side of the volcano are continually reduced. Eventually, the task proves impossible to complete.

Rules for how the game is organized and played promote a range of positive outcomes by:

- structuring cooperation with people with whom one might not otherwise play and thus creating networks of people who work together to achieve a common goal
- eliminating the dichotomy of winners and losers that can easily teach lessons about jealousy, revenge, and protection of image and reputation
- the simple device of requiring physical contact between participants that is supportive rather than confrontational
- demonstrating that it is possible for achievement to take place outside the parameters of a zero-sum game—every

group playing Crossing the Volcano can succeed without having to require other groups to fail

- showing that even with limited resources, it is possible to share in a way that lets everyone achieve
- demonstrating that for a group to be successful (and hence safe and healthy), individuals must act with care not only for themselves, but for others as well

In debriefing after the game, participants soon realize how an activity like this demonstrates important life skills. The success of the game relies on everyone's cooperation and use of effective communication skills. Leaving one person behind results in failure for the rest of the group. Hence, a sense of community building can be taught in a way that is relevant and real to participants. Other skills such as problem solving and critical thinking emerge as the challenges of the task become progressively more difficult. The benefit of developing innovative and creative solutions in situations where resources are scarce becomes evident to the learners.

Using life skills as the roots for an enriched discussion about health, students are then taken on a journey of discovery by a health-minded teacher who uses the game to talk about topics of current interest, such as gender equity, the prevention of HIV/AIDS, the inclusion of children with disabilities, and peaceful conflict resolution. Playing the game encourages students to discover the virtues of thinking first before taking physical action, and of planning for possible consequences before committing to a course of action whose outcomes, like those of violence, must be considered in both the short and long terms. Learning that the loss of a single member of the group to the volcano even though everyone else makes it safely across is an unsuccessful journey despite its apparent success can be, in utilitarian ethical terms, a metaphorical lesson about taking care of others while taking care of oneself.

The teaching and learning possibilities inherent in this type of activity are endless. Experiences such as these that actively engage students in the learning process about health provide unlimited scope to allow children and youth to discover their own lessons in the learning process as an alternative to force-feeding or preaching standard mantras about health. ■

> ***When people become autonomous their values become internal. Their purchases and their choice of work begin to reflect their own authentic needs and desires rather than the values imposed on them by advertisers, family, peers and media.*** —Ferguson, 1980, p. 327

The Art of Living

The term "art of living" refers to leading a good life and it is used in philosophy to talk mostly about living a virtuous life. In psychology, the expression is linked to a person's ability to cope with life's ups and downs and to a sense of happiness. It presents a way of thinking about health that pushes beyond accrual models of learning—how much and for how long students learn—to thinking about what kinds and quality of learning take place. Instead of worrying "Did we cover everything?" teachers ask: "Have students become more curious, imaginative, open-minded, uneasy, or aesthetically aroused about the way their life is unfolding?"

Through our acts of health, we see ourselves and the artistry of our lives. The art of living refers to a form of self-direction with a view to living the good life. It seeks to teach a person to achieve the good life that lies within. In other words, part of the study of health should be to help students answer the question "How should I live my life?" The art of living is much more complex than simply learning to read and write. It entails putting that knowledge and skill into action such that something good happens. In the art of living, the person is both the artist and the object of their art.

According to Rawls (1971), a person is one who expresses two criteria: (a) a capacity for making autonomous decisions and (b) a reflective capacity for understanding the place of one's choices and decisions in relation to one's life plans and for considering the relative merits of different choices. If there is a single argument for the inclusion of health as an area of study, it may well be because it contributes to the development of a person—someone who actively cares for self and others. It is this artistry in which we prepare our students to engage as part of their growth and development as individuals and as citizens. It is important for us to be concerned about ourselves and our opportunities. At the same time, however, we must be aware of whether others are also able to achieve the artistry they desire in their lives.

Veenhoven (2000) uses a matrix to depict the art of living:

	Inner Qualities	Outer Qualities
Life Chances	quality of life life-ability of person	live-ability of environment
Life Results	appreciation of life	utility of life

Veenhoven's exploration of the art of living centres on quality of life. He distinguishes a good life through the examination of a person's opportunities for a good life and the good life itself. This difference he refers to as a person's potentiality and actuality: "life-chances" and "life-results." Opportunities and outcomes are related, but they are certainly not the same. Chances can fail to be realized, due to misinformation or bad luck. Conversely, people sometimes make much of their lives despite poor opportunities.

A second difference Veenhoven describes is between "external" and "internal" qualities. In the first case, quality resides in the environment, while in the latter it resides in the individual. Lane (1994) makes this distinction clear by pointing out the differences between "quality of society" and "quality of persons." Likewise, Musschenga (1994) discerns "quality of the conditions for living" as different from "the quality of being human." This distinction is also quite commonly made in public health. External pathogens are distinguished from inner afflictions, and researchers try to identify the mechanisms by which the former produce the latter, and the conditions in which this is more and less likely to influence health. Yet this basic insight is lacking in many social policy discussions. For instance, in discourses on urban renewal, the term "quality-of-life" is used in association with both clean streets and feelings of being at home in the neighbourhood (Veehoven, 2000). Similarly, in schools there is a good deal of discussion about the importance of psychosocial environments and the impact these have on students' feelings of belonging and acceptance as a factor in school affiliation, social bonding, and academic achievement.

Why Health Is Important in Schools

To this point, this chapter has focused primarily upon the importance of individuals taking health seriously in order to enhance their quality of life and the lives of others. But what happens when an entire school takes health seriously?

Links between good health and favourable education outcomes are clear (Brellochs, 1995; Samdal, Nutbeam, Wold, & Kannas, 1998; Symons, Cincelli, James, & Groff, 1997). Children who enjoy good health are more likely to engage whole-heartedly in school community activities, both academic and non-academic (Allensworth, Lawson, Nicholson, & Wyche, 1997), and are more likely to develop into healthy adults around whom healthy communities can be built (WHO, 1998). The need to extend the importance of health to the entire school environment and encourage the whole school community to sustain such initiatives is essential (Wharf Higgins, Gaul, Gibbons, & Van Gyn, 2003).

The school is an important space where a spirit of community, contribution, and care can direct the learning experience. When the health of the school community is a priority, schools can become a place where attention is focused on how individuals can achieve a greater sense of control over their lives, in addition to reinforcing a sense of belonging, affiliation, and attachment to the school and the surrounding community. The school community can serve as an alternative reality to what students may experience or witness outside of school. The role of the school is to draw into question "What is" and to propose "What if?"

Health mindedness helps us think "care"fully about what schools are "good" for. At the heart of thinking about health as an integral part of school life and learning are beliefs about the purpose and value of schools. To be successful, health initiatives must be clearly aligned with the school system's perceived mandate. Schools must prepare students for competent and responsible participation in society. Student learning is much more than the acquisition of encyclopaedic knowledge, pre-digested points of view, facts, and formulas. It implies, rather, becoming a member of a community of practice. The experience and desire to participate in that community may provide a more powerful motive for learning to participate. Belonging requires a person to see themselves as a member of the community, taking responsibility for their personal actions. The learning process implies a change in personal identity. Learning to participate, therefore, is at the same time learning to become a specific person.

What are schools "good" for and how is health inextricably linked to this purpose? Geert ten Dam, professor of education at the University of Amsterdam, the Netherlands, reflects:

> At the centre of efforts to promote health is the person; the development of a certain kind of person rather than a person who knows certain things! (Anderson & Ronson, 2010, p.222).

What are the implications of ten Dam's statement? Importantly, in addition to acquiring knowledge and skills within a particular field of understanding, students must also consider how this knowledge and set of skills are applied with care in mind—care for self, others, the environment, and significant social issues such as human rights. In other words, students should be encouraged to develop knowledge and skills for the sake of both personal and public "good."

Health and learning are interdependent. Just as health exerts a powerful influence on children's ability to learn, educational achievement is an important determinant of health. Students who are well-adjusted in school are more likely to enjoy school life, engage in post-secondary studies, "have good relationships with their parents, …be healthy and happy, and ... avoid health risk behaviours" (King, Boyce, & King, p. xiii, 1999). A good education can improve an individual's chances of attaining fulfilling and stable employment and, thus, enjoy higher standards of living and, ultimately, enjoy better health through better housing, better health-care products, better food, more stable family life, and greater access to leisure and recreational pursuits (Stephens & Graham, 1993).

However, if we take ten Dam's advice, for education to fulfill its mandate, it should contribute to the overall development of a person. Health and learning are interdependent in that the practice of good health entails involvement in a process of learning that results in the construction of knowledge and the activation of talents and imagination to achieve valued outcomes. In other words, education is healthy when it concentrates on putting knowledge and skills to "good" use. Nussbaum (1990) argues that putting knowledge to good use or practical reasoning is linked directly to the human desire for affiliation (that is, to have concern for other humans, to live for others, and to have familial and other interactions and attachments). Nussbaum contends that the capacity for practical reasoning and affiliation are paramount to the process of education for and through health because everything a person does is planned and organized by her/his ability to reason and is done with concern for self and other humans in mind. In short, a good education prepares us physically, mentally, emotionally, socially, and spiritually to care for self and others.

"If you want improvement, don't treat people as they are, treat them as they are capable of becoming!"—Author unknown.

Health includes feelings of belonging and connectedness. According to Wilkinson (1996), the more disempowered, alienated, and silenced people feel in relation to society, and especially their immediate world—local community affairs, faith community, schools, health-care services, employment services and opportunities—the more likely they are to develop social anxiety, resulting in shame, lowered self-esteem, and feelings of hopelessness and worthlessness. These factors often lead to intense and persistent levels of stress, aggression, depression, substance abuse, and crime.

The gap between the "haves" and the "have-nots" can be a strong indicator of not only social and economic disparities but also disparities in health. The richest societies do not have the best health; rather, it is in societies that have the smallest income differentiation between rich and poor. In a chapter titled "How Society Kills," Wilkinson (1996) presents a large amount of worldwide evidence, stating that, on average, poor people die at an earlier age. This occurs not just for the obvious reasons such as lack of food or exposure to danger. In reality, it is the "psychosocial pathway" that does the most harm. In Wilkinson's words:

> To feel depressed, cheated, bitter, desperate, vulnerable, frightened, angry, worried about debts, or job and housing insecurity; to feel devalued, useless, helpless, uncared for, hopeless, isolated, anxious and a failure; these feelings can dominate people's whole experience of life, coloring their experience of everything else. It is the chronic stress arising from feelings like these, which does the damage. It is the social feelings which matter, not exposure to a supposedly toxic material environment. The material environment is merely the indelible mark and constant reminder of the oppressive fact of one's failure, of the atrophy of any sense of having a place in a community, and of one's social exclusion and devaluation as a human being. (Wilkinson, 1996, p.215)

In other words, prolonged stress damages health. More bluntly, poverty makes you sick. Greater equality in terms of social cohesion is the psychosocial pathway to reducing stress and building a better life. Fewer supportive relationships are associated with poorer health—not just the absence of friends and close relatives, but also "less involvement in wider social networks, community activities, etc." (Wilkinson, 1996, p.182). Therefore, the task for society as a whole must be to facilitate and enrich a sense of belonging and togetherness.

Schools play an important role in helping communities to thrive because they can help develop citizens who care. Healthy children care about other people's feelings: who gets to be involved in activities and who happens to be left out. Healthy learners believe that everyone has the right to enjoy life. Health is about optimizing access to and hope for a better life.

Andy Anderson frequently recounted examples of young children learning to show care and concern for others. One boy found out that children in foster homes in his community carried their belongings in a garbage bag. He launched a campaign to gather suitable luggage for these children because he believed they deserved to have their things respected as well. Another student in Grade 2 named Zoe commented in an editorial published in the *Stratford Beacon Herald*:

> "One thing I do is grow my hair and donate it to Angel Hair for Kids. They make wigs for kids who don't have hair because of things like cancer or if they were in fires. I donated my hair once when I was five and I'm doing it again this month. Angel Hair for Kids needs 12 donations just to make one wig. If you are a hairdresser maybe you can give free haircuts to people who want to send in their hair. These are just my ideas. Maybe when I am older I will have more ideas. It makes me happy to help. Maybe other people will be happy too if they help too."

Health Education as an Integral Part of the Overall Development of Students

Historically, health education in our schools has emphasized healthy habits; disease prevention; behaviour modification, including the benefits of an active lifestyle; and safety and injury prevention. However, an emphasis on individual health, which has often been narrowly defined, has effectively created "boundaries" around the potential of health education to foster healthy school cultures and, through them, healthy communities. This emphasis has perpetuated the separation of health education from the overall school agenda, allowing health literacy to be marginalized as an "add-on." One consequence of the marginalization of health education is that students are put at risk.

Education about health prepares students to cope with challenge and change, to think critically, to resist pressures to engage in unhealthy behaviours, to adopt healthy lifestyle habits, to care about the opportunities others have, and to experience the benefits of healthy living. However, simply teaching children and youth the skills they need to make healthy choices is not enough to ensure that they will apply these skills. They need to be completely supported in making healthy choices. Health education should be viewed as much more than a course of study about specific health topics (such as sexual health or proper nutrition) but rather as an opportunity to foster health mindfulness so that students are supported in every way possible in making healthy choices to benefit themselves and others.

Case Study

By Amanda Stanec

Farnaz is excited about her upcoming move in September when she will begin teaching in a new school within the same school district. With this pending move, Farnaz will decrease her commute from a 45-minute drive each way to having the option to use active transportation with a 5 km commute. During her first three years as a teacher, Farnaz worked tirelessly to help her school progress towards being a health-minded school. She is very proud of what she has accomplished. Now, however, she is nervous. Will all the progress that she, along with her colleagues, have made in leading health-minded initiatives at her current school disappear when she departs? Will she have to begin at square one in promoting health-mindedness in her new school? Some teachers at the new school have told Farnaz that they do not perceive her future principal to be one to value students' health as a school-wide measureable goal or initiative. Farnaz is feeling a little stressed due to what she has heard, coupled with her understanding that there are no school-wide health goals at her new school and that a perception prevails that health is currently taught only as part of a physical education program that focuses heavily on physical health. The school year is approaching and Farnaz is feeling uneasy about her new school and its new administration—so much so, in fact, that it is hindering her sleep at night.

1 What challenges are presented in this case study? How significant are they? Do you think you could solve these challenges easily? On your own? With others?
2 Put yourself in Farnaz's shoes. What personal assets (such as leadership and organizational skills, prior work experience) would you bring to help navigate these challenges? Why do you think these personal assets would be helpful? Have you applied these assets in other instances in which they have served you well? If so, what results did you achieve?
3 What external assets (such as facilities, personnel, and policies) could help you navigate these challenges? Have you relied on any of these assets in the past to help you overcome challenges? Are there any external assets that you normally would not access? If so, why not?
4 Referring to content in this chapter, construct a conversation with the principal at Farnaz's new school in which you present a clear and pertinent rationale and evidence for the benefits of health and health-promoting schools.
5 How would you assess your decisions to determine if they were effective? Do you consider yourself to be a reflective educator? If so, has this served you well in the past? In what ways? Do you think that education in general would benefit from more reflective practices and policies?

It's Your Turn

Develop short-term and long-term goals, as well as performance measures to track progress, that would allow you to apply content from this chapter to your current pre-service teaching setting or employment setting.

Create an assessment strategy to determine the effectiveness of the goals presented in question 1.

✓ Action Checklist

Individual	Suggested Follow-up
Pre-service Teacher	❑ During practicum placements, seek to learn from those leading health initiatives throughout the school community. ❑ Reflect on your ability to plan, deliver, and assess lessons centred on health mindedness. ❑ Meet with other pre-service teachers to brainstorm ideas and share resources related to health mindedness and health-promoting norms.
Health and Physical Education Teacher	❑ Collaborate closely with other teachers at your school and/or take on a leadership role to create health-promoting norms. ❑ Meet with all those responsible for teaching health and physical education to ensure that (a) there is vertical articulation in the program planning and delivery, and (b) all health outcomes are taught in the most logical way. (Note: often this includes integrated teaching.) ❑ View yourself as a leader and a resource for others and be approachable by others who may want to increase health-promoting norms in the school community. ❑ Educate your colleagues on health mindedness and how they can apply it to develop a healthier school community. ❑ Lead a faculty meeting or school-wide health fair to help create a ripple effect for the development of health-promoting norms throughout the school community.
Administrator	❑ Incorporate health-promoting norms into faculty goal setting. ❑ Encourage optimal health for students and staff.
Parent/Guardian	❑ Ask school administrators about health policies at the district and school levels. ❑ Ask health and physical education teachers about how learning outcomes are being taught, and if they can teach all outcomes to students given the current time mandated in each content area. ❑ Inform your child's school administrator, district superintendent, and school board that you believe that health and physical education is a critical and necessary component of a quality educational experience.

Chapter 1 Summary

Schools are ideally suited not only to prepare children and youth with the skills they need to make healthy choices, but also to serve as the cornerstone for healthy communities. When school communities value health, several educational principles emerge that permeate every aspect of a school's culture.

The primary goal of schools is to optimize learning for active participation in society. The concept of health mindfulness is developed in and through schools to encourage tomorrow's citizens to make decisions and choices with health in mind.

Education and health are inextricably linked. Educational outcomes relate to health status, and health outcomes relate to educational achievement. Healthy children learn better. Higher levels of educational attainment can result in stable and satisfying employment, better problem-solving skills, greater optimism, and a sense of confidence about life chances—all of which are intertwined with better health.

Questions for Reflection

1 As you think about what health means to people and schools, also think metacognitively about the sources of knowledge referenced in exploring these ideas. Where does your way of thinking about healthy living originate? Do you draw upon cultural traditions, family habits and attitudes, or interpretations presented by the medical community, popular media, or advertising industry?

2 How does the school culture invite students to have a hand in addressing health issues? Do students feel they have a say in what they are taught, how they express their understanding of the subject matter, and the degree to which they participate in school governance?

3 Think about your own health as an educator. What might constitute a checkup on your own health? Have you engaged in any kind of systematic inquiry into your own professional practice? For instance, how does an activity break affect your levels of alertness and concentration? Do you invite colleagues to work with you to improve your instructional skills?

4 Think about your own health as a person. Do you make time for personal reflection and spiritual well-being? Do you devote time to helping others? Do you participate in an exercise program: walking, biking, swimming, inline skating, or other activities you enjoy?

5 What happens when people make decisions through a health lens? For example, when buying a new pair of shoes, you might choose a comfortable, all-purpose runner with good support that you could wear while walking or biking to work. Consider how you would think about these everyday choices with health in mind:

- buying a new or used car
- hosting a birthday party
- upgrading your bathroom
- planning a summer excursion

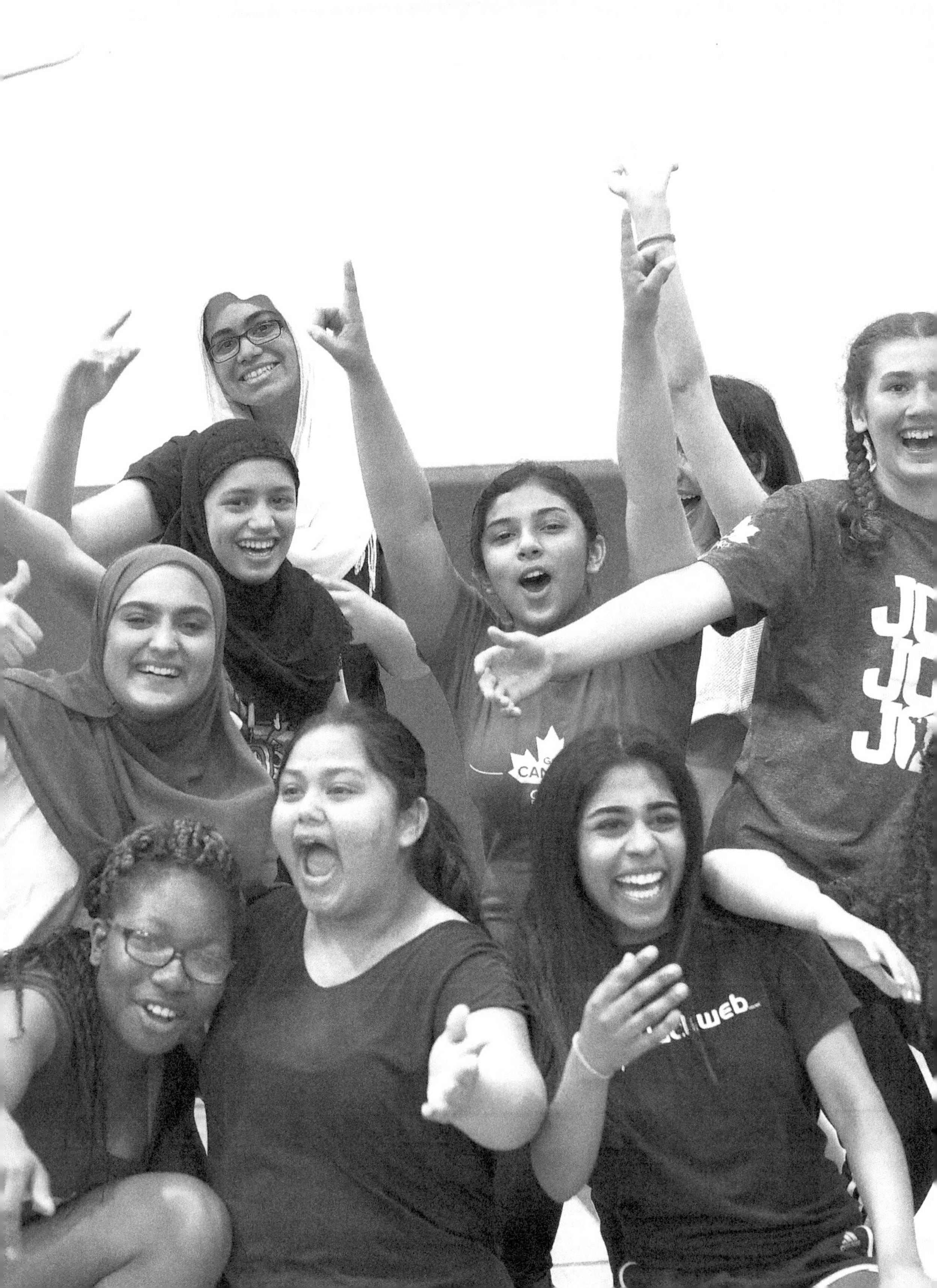

2

Health-Promoting Schools

Optimizing opportunities for everyone

One of the most highly regarded and successful international educational endeavours is captured in the idea of the health-promoting school. WHO (1998) defines a health-promoting school (HPS) as "a school that is constantly strengthening its capacity as a healthy setting for living, learning, and working." In partnership with a range of human service providers, health-promoting schools aim to provide the means, conditions, and environments that optimize opportunities for both students and teachers to learn. Underlying the concept of health promotion is the notion that to achieve good health, people must exercise agency or at least some measure of control over the decisions and conditions they encounter in their lives over time and across circumstances.

The following section describing the features of health-promoting schools represents an amalgamation of ideas presented in three articles co-authored by Andy Anderson.[1]

1 The majority of the following section was published previously by the lead author. See Anderson, Andy. (2005). Understanding school improvement and school effectiveness from a health promoting school perspective. REICE. *Revista Iberoamericana sobre Calidad, Eficacia y Cambio en Educación*, 282–296.

What Is a Health-Promoting School?

Contemporary notions of health that cast humans as constructivists and creators who can exercise determination over their own well-being focus on building within people a capacity to "make a life" by enhancing their ability to learn—that is, to cope, adapt, and make sense of their environments and relationships. Health promotion is defined as "the process of enabling people to increase control over and to improve their health. To reach a state of complete physical, mental, and social wellbeing, an individual or group must be able to identify and to realize aspirations, to satisfy needs, and to change and to cope with the environment" (WHO—Ottawa Charter, 1986).

The European Network of Health Promoting Schools, supported jointly by WHO, the Council of Europe, and the European Union, consists of approximately 500 schools from 41 countries. It reaches about 10 thousand teachers and half a million students. In Canada and the United States, the conceptual roots of health promotion in school settings date to the 1980s when there arose a strong call for continuous "comprehensive school health" (CSH) education from kindergarten to graduation. Early proponents of CSH argued that health habits and knowledge acquired early in life could impact lifelong health status. Health education portrayed simply as a course of study was considered ineffective. Rather, the overall curriculum could be part of school-wide and community efforts to promote healthy living. And the curriculum for health education might address a wide array of topics every year that developmentally build the skills and habits of mind needed to cope with divergent needs and evolving circumstances related to health literacy and well-being. Health education, like other subjects offered in school, should ideally prepare young people to be lifelong, autonomous, and responsible learners and as such represents an important area of study related to human development.

Subsequently, comprehensive health programs sought to facilitate health services and school environments—hallways, playgrounds, gymnasiums, cafeterias, and so on—that were considered equally important for students' health. Perhaps a classic example of incongruence between health education and school environments has been the tension between nutrition education aimed at promoting healthy food choices and the sale of junk food in vending machines and school fundraising campaigns. Unless a school is committed to healthy eating and healthy food options, the effects of the health-education program can be undermined.

Clearly, responsibility for health promotion has been broadened and enriched to involve a wide spectrum of services and supports. In a health-promoting school, student learning, effective teaching practices, and school improvement plans are guided, inspired, and nurtured through a health-promotion lens. Thus, teachers can address the physical, mental, social-emotional, and spiritual factors that influence student learning. The result is a school environment in which students feel that they belong, in which they feel safe, and in which they are invited to participate in decisions that affect their opportunities for learning and leadership.

At the heart of each school health-promotion model are several principles that serve as a moral compass for decisions about the purpose, structure, and engagement of people within organizations, institutions, and programs of study. These ten principles were first adopted in 1997 by resolution at the first conference of the European Network of Health Promoting Schools. These principles are central to campaigns for health promotion in schools and they highlight fundamental rights and entitlements for children and youth that underpin the formation of a just and civil society. These enduring principles have been translated into several languages since their adoption:

- Democracy—giving children voice and choice. In democratic learning environments, students are encouraged to express their ideas and to listen to alternative points of view.
- Equity—different ways of knowing and showing what you know. Healthy schools foster the emotional and social development of every individual and provide access to a full range of educational opportunities.
- Empowerment and action competence—what can you give? Health-promoting schools improve young people's abilities to take action, cope with challenges, and generate change. When youth are empowered because of new ideas and visions, they can better direct their life course and ultimate living conditions.
- Collaboration—we are all in this together. Sharing responsibility and resources is a central part of strategic planning.
- Communities mean that two heads are better than one. Working in partnership represents a powerful force for positive change.
- Curriculum—a healthy school's curriculum provides opportunities for young people to gain knowledge and insight and to acquire essential life skills. Curriculum must be relevant to the needs of young people both now and in the future. It must stimulate creativity, encourage learning, and provide students with essential skills. The curriculum can also be a stimulus to the personal and professional development of teachers and others employed by the school.
- Teacher development—invest in teacher learning. Teachers are learners, too.
- Sustainability—there are no quick fixes. Commit resources to long-term sustainable development.
- Measure success—how do we know whether change occurs unless we determine where we started and where we are now? Assessment is an integral part of instruction and planning. Make sure to assess process and outcomes!
- The school environment. The physical characteristics and social culture of the school have a profound effect on health.

These principles recognize schools as a key setting for health promotion because schools can provide universal access to knowledge, skills, services, and supports, thus building within individuals and communities a capacity for change agency and growth. Furthermore, health promotion "works" when it is aligned systematically and consistently with the goals and mandates of the organization in which it is presented. School experiences managed in relation to these principles are posed as a way to broaden and intensify students' involvement in what Habermas (1990) has termed the "lifeworld" of schools: cultural traditions, ceremonial rituals, participation in clubs, and teacher-student relationships; as well as the "systems world" of schools: programs of study and school governance. Authentic involvement in school life can build feelings of affiliation and connectedness. Enriched student participation builds trust; greater awareness of students' needs, interests, talents, values, and goals; and mutual understanding between teachers and students. When students feel that they are heard, respected, and have a say, they are more likely to contribute to and comply with school mandates. In other words, following health-promotion principles such as a regard for democracy can be viewed as a way to make schools stronger and healthier.

The health-promoting school is also celebrated as a way to forge stronger links between the community—the local cultural context and customs—and approaches to health promotion. In this way, health promotion builds on resources unique to each school community. Community characteristics are viewed as assets to be developed, not problems to be overcome. Lerner and Benson's *Developmental Assets and Asset-Building Communities* (2003) provides a review of programs and research that make a convincing argument for the notion of growth and change in relation to community resources—most importantly, a community's strengths, imagination, hopes, and dreams. Increasingly, community service groups are taking up this challenge through initiatives such as the Lions Quest program of Lions Clubs International. Operating in more than 50 countries, including Canada and the United States, Lions Quest promotes the positive social-emotional development of students. The program focuses on positive behaviours; connection to school; anti-bullying; character education; learning about service provision; and drug, alcohol, and tobacco awareness. Programs that activate community involvement and integrate the principles of health promotion enable schools to get smarter in identifying the specific needs and opportunities that exist within their local communities.

School environments that work to respect everyone's right to enjoy school attendance, share ideas and insights openly, challenge the status quo, and question existing practices and power relationships foster rich opportunities for critical and alternative thinking. Under these conditions, schools become safe and healthy havens for everyone.

As an integral part of overall efforts to improve schools for "public" good (that is, the betterment of society, responsible citizenry, and care for self and others), a health-promoting school is conceptually represented as:

- A stance or disposition toward learning. openness to ideas; respect for alternative views and realities; and acknowledgement of learning as a social process linked to time, place, and context
- A way of being in the classroom, community, or world. actively pursuing meaning from multiple texts, and protecting and promoting opportunities for everyone to learn by creating environments that are inviting and safe

- A way of belonging. relating learning to citizenry and contribution to the betterment of society, and relating knowing and doing to community participation—communities of scholarship and communities of care;
- An organizational model. how people, programs, policy, and partners interrelate and work together in relation to common values and principles such as equity and empowerment (Anderson & Ronson, 2010)

The health-promoting school model also increases awareness of how societal values impact all health-related activity. For example, peace, social justice, reducing the educational and economic inequities associated with low income and unemployment, and enhancing the social capital that affords meaningful engagement in civic and social life are inextricably linked to health and social problems.

Health-Promoting Schools as a Comprehensive Approach to Health

School health promotion uses the school setting to promote the health of students, staff, and the community as part of a community-wide population health approach.[2] "Comprehensive" as an adjective attached to health promotion often causes confusion. It is meant to emphasize that health promotion should take into account a wide range of factors and influences. Ideally, health promotion should be:

(a) Holistic. encompass the mental, physical, social, spiritual, and environmental well-being of all persons

(b) Multi-layered. involve all layers of influence on schools (students, parents or guardians, teachers, vice-principals, principals, support staff, and government officials)

(c) Multi-sector. involve all sectors that influence opportunities to learn, e.g., employment, transportation, environmental care, health services, economic development, and so on

(d) Multidisciplinary. involve all areas of curriculum and scholarship (e.g., economics, labour, feminism, history, geography, and so on)

According to the Pan-Canadian Joint Consortium on School Health (JCSH, 2005), comprehensive school health includes a broad spectrum of programs, activities, and services that take place in schools and their surrounding communities. The goals of these programs, activities, and services are to enable children and youth to enhance their health, develop their fullest potential, and establish productive and satisfying relationships in their lives. The approach is designed to affect not only individual health behaviours, but also to improve the environments in which young people live and learn (McCall, 1999, p.4). To improve the health of our students, educators must think both in terms of the curriculum and in terms of the larger school and social contexts.

The programs, activities, and services delivered within such comprehensive approaches to school health involve the committed participation of young people, families, professionals, institutions, agencies, and organizations concerned with children and

---

2 This section has been reused with permission from: Canadian Association for School Health and Others (2007). *Canadian Consensus Statement on Comprehensive School Health* (Revised Edition), Surrey, BC. The lead author, Andy Anderson, was a contributor to the development of this document.

youth, education, health, social services, law enforcement, the voluntary sector, and the community as well as governments at all levels. Each of these individuals, organizations, and government departments can potentially augment the delivery of instruction, services, social support, or a healthy physical environment. Effective school-based health promotion uses comprehensive approaches that:

- integrate our responses to health issues within a holistic view of health and the whole child
- favour values such as youth engagement, parent involvement, and staff wellness
- coordinate multiple interventions at all levels within several systems and agencies that serve children and youth and that result in health-promoting school communities

Collectively, the goals of comprehensive school health approaches are to:

- promote health and wellness
- prevent diseases, disorders, and injury
- intervene to assist children and youth who are in need or at risk
- support those who are already experiencing poor health
- provide an equitable playing field that addresses disparities and contributes to academic success

Experience and research evidence strongly suggest that a comprehensive approach to school-based and school-linked health promotion can influence the health-related knowledge, attitudes, and behaviours of students, as well as modify or alleviate other factors that compromise health (Murray, Low, Hollis, Cross, & Davis, 2007).

Expectations regarding the impact of the school setting must be realistic, however, because the primary determinants of health status (family expectations and practices; developmental issues; genetics; and socio-economic, cultural, and environmental factors) exert a profound impact.

The Four Pillars of Comprehensive School Health

> ***"Comprehensive School Health is an integrated approach to health promotion that gives students numerous opportunities to observe and learn positive health attitudes and behaviours. It aims to reinforce health consistently on many levels and in many ways."*** —Public Health Agency of Canada, 2007

The JCSH comprehensive school health framework has four pillars: 1) teaching and learning; 2) partnerships and services; 3) social and physical environment; and 4) policy. According to Bassett-Gunter, Yessis, Manske, and Gleddie (2015), "when actions in all four pillars are harmonised, students are supported to realize their full potential as learners and as healthy, productive members of society" (p. 239).

The JCSH Comprehensive School Health Framework

Teaching and Learning

- a comprehensive, K-12 health curriculum; K-12 physical education curriculum; family studies program
- the integration of health into other subject areas
- the planned use of other informal learning opportunities
- the development of awareness, knowledge, attitudinal change, decision making, skill building, behavioural change, and social responsibility
- effective pre-service and in-service training for educators
- appropriate teaching methodologies that are culturally and developmentally sensitive, including use of the Internet and other media

Partnerships and Services

- role modelling by school staff and others
- peer support
- media cooperation
- community participation
- staff wellness programs
- effective school management practices
- active student participation
- extensive parental involvement

Social and Physical Environment

- bully-free and anti-violence school policies
- coordinated support services among school, home, and community
- school mission and vision statements to support psychological and social health of the school community
- positive health role models
- peer support programs
- a positive school climate and ethos

Policy

- safety procedures and regulations
- sanitation, clean water
- environmental health standards
- healthy food and nutrition policies and services
- smoke-free school policies
- accessible and sustainable environments that promote safety and freedom from bullying or harassment

Not all communities, agencies, governments, or sectors will accept all the components or aspects of a comprehensive approach to school health programs. However, it is vitally important that constituents at every level and in each sector take ownership for school health promotion and ensure that the strategies used are relevant to the local customs, cultures, and traditions of the school community. This requires that they embrace the opportunity and obligation to develop their own approach, define their own models, and select their own priorities consistent with the resources available to them.

The Role of Policy in Creating and Supporting Health-Promoting Schools

Just as dedicated and forward-thinking teachers serve as change-inducing role models, comprehensive and forward-thinking school policies at multiple levels can play a key role in effecting positive, health-promoting change throughout schools, boards, and regions.

The JCHS definition of *healthy school policy,* which includes management practices, decision-making processes, and rules and procedures at all levels of education, is clear evidence that policies are a primary foundation for the creation and support of healthy school communities.

"Healthy School Communities in Canada" (Bassett-Gunter, Yessis, Manske & Gleddie, 2015) synthesizes and clarifies key concepts across jurisdictions and proposes a common understanding of healthy school communities. Policy clearly emerges as a critical cross-jurisdictional priority regardless of local vocabulary or nuance. The paper identifies five fundamental principles of the healthy school approach. Policy is embedded in each principle:

1 **Whole school approach.** "This approach incorporates a healthy culture through structures, policies and procedures for staff, students and community to model and promote health and well-being" (p.7).

2 **Education and health synergy.** "Joint planning and coordinating policies and resources (e.g., funding, time) across the health and education sectors can reduce duplication of efforts to enhance student well-being and decrease gaps in existing policies and practices" (p.7).

3 **Leadership team/committed champions.** "...engaging a team of individuals with strong commitment, relationships (JCSH, 2008), communication and management practices will aid in facilitating healthy school community actions" (p.8).

4 **Assessment, planning, and evaluation.** "...school communities should assess ... existing resources including their current healthy school community actions, policies, goals, structures, resources..." (p.8).

5 **Planning for sustainability.** "...there must be long-term anchoring of the healthy school community initiatives into policy at the school and district levels" (p.8).

SUCCESS STORY

Aquatic Lifesaving in the Caribbean

By Andy Anderson

A group of student teachers in the Caribbean initiated a unit of study on aquatic lifesaving by brainstorming to identify the many different people who, as part of their careers, are interested in the various aspects of lifesaving. Their list included, for example, lifeguards, members of the coast guard, oceanographers, nurses, doctors, emergency medical and rescue personnel, and hotel pool designers. They then connected each area of interest to subject matter study and key questions.

1 What are the mechanics of swimming, for example, swim strokes, drown-proofing, buoyancy? (physics, mathematics)
2 What causes tides and riptides? (geography and oceanography)
3 What is artificial respiration? (physiology of respiration)
4 What skills are needed to serve as a rescuer or lifeguard coast guard member? (mathematics, map reading, physical fitness)
5 How should swimming pools be designed to maximize observation by parents and lifeguards, and reduce the incidence of accident and injury? (mathematics, architecture, and visual arts)
6 What do parents need to know to ensure that children are safe in the water? (language and visual arts, media literacy, drama)

Exploring health issues through the integration of knowledge from other subject areas is not only an integral part of a health-promoting school, but also an effective way to foster learning and understanding in general. Students applied research and reporting skills to an important health concern on the island, as very few children and adults learn how to swim. Despite the widespread lack of swimming skills, it is important to learn lifesaving skills since many people earn their living from the sea.

Subject-area integration enabled teachers to bring knowledge to bear on a critical issue and make evident the importance of knowledge acquisition beyond test taking. Students could also become engaged in discussions about how knowledge from different perspectives contributes to their overall understanding of a topic.

Among the most powerful dimensions were the stories students told of relatives or friends who had lost their lives due to drowning and the grief and sense of loss that remained long after the incident. People's everyday lives are touched by these tragedies. Although much of the harm avoidance practices seem mechanical, they are linked directly to feelings of care for self and others.

The study powerfully illustrates that at the heart of integration is the notion that learning is for life—lifelong learning, making life better and helping others enjoy a good life. ■

Examples of Healthy School Policies

Ecological systems theory (Bronfenbrenner, 2005; Bronfenbrenner & Morris, 1998) postulates that interrelated yet distinct systems affect human behaviour. This theory suggests that individuals interact within multiple levels of human ecological systems, ranging from proximal microsystems to more distal macrosystems. Ecological systems theory offers a broad framework for viewing the various levels and interconnectedness of aspects of policy as evidenced in health-promoting schools. Here are examples of how policy is implemented at different levels.

- Classroom level. Policies at this level can be as simple as allowing water bottles on desks or as complex as setting out rules and guidelines for students' behaviour toward one other (social-emotional environment). Classroom policies also give teachers the flexibility to make decisions such as allowing students to work at a stand-up desk or allowing only healthy treats and prizes.
- School level. Schools can adopt policies ranging from how students are treated (anti-bullying policies), to the kinds of physical activities (intramurals, school sports) that are offered, to the types of food that are allowed in vending machines.
- District level. Authorities at the district level exercise a mandate to declare and implement policies that each school must follow. For example, in the Battle River School District in Alberta, Policy 21, titled Healthy School Communities and Workplaces, formalizes the importance of student and staff wellness (Gleddie, 2012).
- Provincial level. In Canada, education is the responsibility of provincial governments. Therefore, this is the "highest" level of policy creation. Curriculum is an example of policy at this level. Other examples are the Daily Physical Activity (DPA) policies implemented in Alberta, Ontario, and British Columbia.
- National/international level. Policy guidelines and recommendations such as WHO's Regional Guidelines for the Development of Health-Promoting Schools, although not enforceable, are important advocacy documents that can help provide structure and direction at a provincial level. Another example is the widely influential UNESCO Quality Physical Education Policy Project that provides tools, graphics, and information for educational jurisdictions to use or adapt to their own purposes (www.unesco.org).

Assessing Healthy School Policies

There are several informal ways to assess the efficacy of the policies related to promoting a healthy school community:

- Survey teachers, students, parents and guardians, and community members (using simple tools such as Survey Monkey, for example, that provide excellent graphics) on a variety of topics, including their understanding of policy. Be sure to share results with the school community so as to fill any knowledge gaps and inform partnership action plans.

- Conduct interviews with key partners and/or those stakeholders who are most affected by policies and procedures at both the school and board levels.
- Host informal focus groups consisting of a cross-section of members of your school community to invite feedback on new ideas, policies, or directions.
- Invite school community members to regular discussion sessions to generate new ideas, provide input, and look to the future.
- Access mechanisms that already exist, such as parent councils, staff meetings, student leadership clubs, and other groups or forums to pose questions about how members of the school community perceive the effectiveness of policies operating at various levels.

The JCSH has also developed a formal assessment protocol called the Healthy School Planner. This easy-to-use resource consists of a variety of tools to help assess the overall school environment. An assessment begins with a foundational module that examines the following:

- Forming your team. Who is involved? Who needs to be involved?
- Planning. Do you use data to make decisions? Do you set goals?
- Implementation across the four pillars. What does implementation look like in each of the following: physical and social environment; healthy school policy; partnerships and services; and teaching and learning?
- Celebrating. How often does your school celebrate healthy school initiatives?
- Sustaining. Do you have a leadership succession plan in place?
- Monitoring and evaluation. How often and by what means do you assess progress?

Using the Healthy School Planner, school teams can access either an "express" or "detailed" set of modules to assess healthy eating, physical activity, positive mental health, and reduction of tobacco use. Completing the HSP can help a school community take stock of its resources, needs, priorities, liabilities, and potential community partnerships (including amenities, fundraising, training, and expertise); weigh recommendations for improvement or amelioration; and finally, devise an action plan related to health promotion.

Given the national scope of the JCSH Comprehensive School Health framework and its recognition by WHO and other international organizations, this framework serves as the foundation for the discussion of healthy schools in this book. The policy dimension of the framework helps shape the other three pillars that support a health-promoting school. Chapters 3 to 7 provide a detailed and comprehensive overview of these pillars. **Chapter 3** focuses on how effective teaching and learning are critical to fostering a health-promoting school. In particular, it underscores the importance of confident and competent teachers in delivering effective curriculum not only in terms of health education, but also in terms of integration of health concepts into other curricular subjects. **Chapter 4** highlights the important role of the physical environment in helping to create and sustain a healthy school. **Chapter 5** identifies the key social supports needed to promote positive social, emotional, and mental health. Finally, **Chapter 6** shines a light on the people who provide important partnerships and services within the school community and thus play important roles in creating a safe, warm, and welcoming healthy school environment. **Chapter 7** contains a number of examples at local, provincial, national, and international levels of how the elements of a healthy school can be implemented in schools and communities around the world.

The Benefits of Health-Promoting Schools

The need to extend the health paradigm to the entire school environment and encourage the whole school community to sustain such initiatives is critical (Wharf Higgins, Gaul, Gibbons, & Van Gyn, 2003). The links between good health and favourable education outcomes are clear. In a comprehensive review, Suhrcke and Nieves (2011) reported that "child health status positively affects educational performance and attainment" (p. vi). Children who enjoy good health are more likely to engage whole-heartedly in school community activities, both academic and non-academic (Allensworth et al., 1997), and are more likely to develop into healthy adults upon whom healthy communities can be built (WHO, 1998). The attainment of these health goals will contribute to more effective schooling, higher academic achievement, and enhanced equity in educational outcomes. When effectively implemented, health-promoting schools can enable children and youth to enhance their health, to learn and develop to their fullest potential, and to establish productive and satisfying relationships in their present and future lives. A wide range of government-sponsored health-promotion and social-development programs may be supported by health-promoting school communities. Ultimately, the comprehensive school health approach can reduce or defer the costs of health care and other human services.[3]

Approaches May Vary but Not Compete

There are several effective approaches to school-based and school-linked health promotion. When implementing a health-promoting schools approach, the JCSH (McCall & Andrew, 2006) provides several worthwhile recommendations:

- The approach can focus on specific health or social issues one at a time, or on three or four issues at a time as they arise. The single-issue approach can use a coordinated strategy by delivering multiple interventions simultaneously.
- The approach can be a sub-population approach (focusing on high-risk students, students living in poverty, gender, culture, Indigenous students, and so on).
- The approach can be based on a type of intervention (e.g., a focus on improving instruction or type of instruction such as skills-based instruction or active learning, development of health services, strengthening of youth participation, development of staff skills, and so on).

3 This section has been reused with permission from: Canadian Association for School Health and Others (2007). *Canadian Consensus Statement on Comprehensive School Health (Revised Edition)*, Surrey, BC.

- The approach can be values-driven, promoting universal principles such as equity, human rights, youth participation, parent involvement, democracy, community development, and social cohesion.
- The approach can be driven by learning and educational objectives and can seek improvements in health and social development so that schools become more effective and simultaneously seek their own improvement.
- The approach can combine specific health issues in an ad-hoc way, based on available resources and expediency.
- The approach can combine health issues under two categories: chronic and communicable diseases.
- The health issues can be grouped under a youth risk/behaviour approach to focus on topics such as smoking, drinking, using drugs, taking sexual risks, or risking injury.
- The approach can focus on life or social skills, social influences, social/emotional development, and mental health to support positive behaviours and prevent or reduce negative health and social behaviours.
- The approach to healthy child and adolescent development as well as health risks and behaviours can seek to modify the key social and physical environments (homes, schools, and communities) that influence these behaviours and development.
- A comprehensive approach combines changes in individual behaviours, skills, knowledge, and attitudes as well as modifications to environments, conditions, and services.
- A comprehensive approach can be pursued through a systems-based methodology that develops certain capacities within the systems, including coordinated policy/leadership, staffing dedicated to school health coordination, formal and informal mechanisms for cooperation, knowledge exchange, sustained workforce development, early identification of emerging issues, and surveillance of health/monitoring of system capacity.

Critical Factors in Creating Healthy Schools

The implementation approaches that the JCSH describes are supported by Bassett-Gunter et al. (2015), who conducted a pan-Canadian review of successful healthy school programs. Their research identified five fundamental principles for successful implementation:

1 Create a whole-school approach that involves and engages all members of the school community.

2 Integrate education and health policies within the school. For example, to support healthy nutrition education, many schools have passed policies prohibiting the sale of drinks with a high sugar content within the school.

3 While healthy schools should strive toward engaging all members of the school community, it is important to appoint a champion or a small group of leaders who will provide oversight, advocacy, and guidance to ensure successful implementation.

4 Use of formative assessments and evaluations to help identify areas of success and areas needing improvement. These assessment and evaluation tools should specifically measure the targeted outcomes that are unique and essential to a specific healthy school community.

5 To be truly successful, a school health program should be sustainable over a long period of time. One-off programs organized once are less effective than initiatives that last throughout the year and that continually grow and develop year after year.

Why All Educators Should Value School-Based Health Promotion

Unless all educators value health promotion, it will remain the purview of health educators. As such, educators will think of health primarily as a course of study, a set of learning outcomes, or a credit to be earned. Health as a resource for living and learning offers a school community much more. Educators who view health promotion as a platform from which to develop the skills and dispositions associated with lifelong learning, the practical application of knowledge, and the transformational experience of learning incorporate health into all aspects of school life. For these educators and their students, health is not an add-on. Rather, it serves as a foundation for all learning.

Health optimizes learning. Children who are sick, tired, and afraid have difficulty learning. Readiness for learning through health promotion can involve everything from a good night's sleep, to feelings of being cared for and having someone to care about, to appropriate eyewear for reading, to participation in clubs at school where young people can interact positively.

Health promotes intellectual character. The study of health topics and issues provides a rich opportunity to develop the habits of mind (ethical reasoning, critical thinking, and action planning) associated with the overall well-being of self and others. A close look at health concerns (e.g., bullying, poverty, violence, pollution, and human sexuality) can engage students deeply in the thinking and doing that are integral parts of active citizenry, social change, and human rights advocacy.

Health promotion develops action competence. Practical reasoning and a capacity for affiliation comprise the fundamental qualities of character and association needed for health and wellbeing. Health promotion is concerned with doing the things that improve health and the conditions that support it; therefore, health is really about taking action—engaging in the "practice of health." Students engaged in the study of health-related issues must be prepared to take on enterprising new roles that involve the use of learning strategies, in addition to communication and inquiry skills similar to those applied in real-world situations.

Linking academic knowledge to health issues is a way for students to relate what they are learning to the complexities of daily living. Health is a way to make learning vivid and real. As but one example, students might calculate the amount and types of garbage disposed in and around the school. In response to their findings, they can devise ways to encourage recycling and waste-reducing alternative food choices on the part of every member of the school community.

The action competence learning process provides a framework by which students can take individual or collective action in response to an important health issue. The term "action competence" means the development of those competencies (understandings and skills) that enable students to take critical action. Together, key stakeholders work together throughout a process to not only identify an area of "action," but to also work together throughout the entire process to critically and creatively plan, implement, and evaluate the process on an ongoing basis (Tasker, 2000). Assuming that education should prepare young people for active participation in society, it seems reasonable and indeed responsible for educators to consciously involve students in dealing with contemporary social, political, and economic issues. Young people want to have a say and a hand in the activities that directly affect their lives. An action competence orientation to learning makes overt the notion that knowing and doing and valuing must be linked. The issue selected for action should be one that students have chosen so that it has meaning and relevance for them. Issues will emerge out of the themes or contexts that are studied. For example, how should a school's physical education program be organized to promote inclusive learning experiences that take the needs, preferences, and capabilities of all students into account? Or how can we encourage all our students and teachers to make choices that ensure healthy, active living?

Through action competence learning, students engage in creative thinking to visualize how things could be or to decide what improvements they would like to see. They analyze an issue and their responses to it to determine what is possible, and then proceed to identify what could help them achieve their goal (enablers) and what could hinder them (barriers). They develop a plan of action and implement it. After completing an action, students evaluate the outcome(s) and identify what they have learned from the experience (even if their original goal has not been achieved). The evaluation may reveal that there are significant environmental or social factors that need to be addressed before a goal can be realized. If this is the case, they begin the process again (Tasker, 2002).

Health promotion humanizes learning. Health as an integral part of the learning process adds care for self and others to the teaching/learning process and to school improvement. Thinking about subject-matter knowledge in relation to care for self and others adds a moral and ethical dimension to the purposes of learning. Health-minded educators plan instruction by asking: "What 'good' is it to know this course material?" "What are schools 'good' for?" In other words, how can life at school and course content contribute to the optimization of students' life chances?

To care and be cared for are fundamental human needs linked to health behaviour. In order to care for someone or something, a sense of the other must be understood, received, respected, and recognized. Health can be a zone where knowledge and skills are applied to problems or issues in such a way as to reveal the value of knowing in relation to improvements in the quality of life of others around us. Health helps educators humanize learning.

Learning with concern for health prepares students to think critically, reason responsibly, imagine possibilities, create alternative solutions, and anticipate consequences such that "good" things will happen. Some of the ways in which schools integrate health are amazingly simple; some are tremendously complex. Each approach creates a context for better learning. For example, a teacher who grows plants in the classroom teaches students about the beauty and biology of plant growth. Furthermore, when experts in horticulture and plant nursery operations collaborate with students, all parties share in a community- and knowledge-building experience that reinforces the importance of plant life and social cooperation.

> ***Where there is life there is hope. In a garden, as indeed on the planet, the miracle of continuing life is cause for the most profound optimism.*** —Goodall (2006, p.56)

Another example of health integration occurs when students, teachers, police, and parents or guardians work together to plan walking routes to school. Mapping safe routes and organizing walking school busses enable children to enjoy walking to school with other students, appreciate the outdoors, and reduce the need for dozens of cars idling outside the main entrance of the school on weekday mornings and afternoons.

Health promotion is about excellence. A health-promoting school is dedicated to excellence in teaching regardless of the subject, to student involvement in the life of the school, and to partnerships with the wider community in order to deepen understanding of local cultures and strengthen the school's relationship with the community at large.

> ***A school cannot be health promoting if it doesn't have in place anti-harassment practices and behaviour management policies. Social justice and equity goals need to be put into practice in the classroom; parent and student participation needs to move beyond parent councils and student representative groups. In essence, health-promoting schools are about sound practice. I view it as an umbrella term for a well-functioning, happy and safe school that aims to educate the whole person.*** —High school principal (New South Wales, Australia).

One School's Health-Promotion Journey

Asked to describe what a health-promoting school meant to them, all the teachers and the principal at one school gave similar responses. One teacher defined a health-promoting school as a "community place that is a nexus of good ideas for all we do; a learning place where we are teaching the kids a lot of concepts that they can apply in their everyday lives." The administrator's definition went deeper. She described a health-promoting school as one that "promotes good health in all we do." In her words:

> Promoting health cannot just be via one route, but instead, it needs to be incorporated in the curriculum and everyday school culture. There always needs to be a wellness component to everything we do here. This school looks at HP from a physical health, happiness and wellness perspective that goes beyond the traditional pathological health definition. Health promotion can't be one person's dream; rather, everyone needs to be involved and be made aware in order for a school to effectively promote health.

A Health and Physical Education teacher at the school identified three major components of a health-promoting school:

- educating students by means of a number of different strategies (that is, multiple intelligences); exhibiting an integrated, multi-level program.
- establishing social networks in the schools (teacher/student, student/student, etc.). These social connections make staff and students feel embedded in the school culture.
- enabling students to participate in a variety of activities ranging from music to drama to physical education. This provides students with an opportunity to explore their unique abilities, interests, and talents. A health-promoting school needs to incorporate health as part of the culture of the school so that it becomes second nature—akin to a common language that is spoken throughout the school.

In collaborative sessions, the entire staff at the school developed the following mission statement:

> *Live, laugh, love, learn in harmony and strive to leave a legacy.*
> (School motto)

The principal further describes the school mission statement in action as follows:

> Everything that takes place at our school fits into this broad enough statement. The word "live" means to be active, to be a leader, to be a driver. "Laugh" means to enjoy your stay at our school by getting involved in your school and remembering to laugh. "Love" is discussed throughout the school as caring for others (those who are less fortunate), caring for oneself, caring for your belongings and the belongings of others and, lastly, caring for the environment. The "learn" component emphasizes learning academically and socially—the goal of education! The harmony component addresses issues of conflict resolution

and peace within the school, the community, and the larger global world. "Leave a legacy behind" encourages students to leave something behind at our school, including a good reputation, an activity you initiated, or simply a smile. This invites students to take pride in their school and make a positive contribution to their school in some way.

The mission statement is simply worded and clear to the students and everyone else in the community. It is displayed throughout the school and shared with parents and guardians via newsletters and other media. The statement is embedded in the school culture and is referred to often during assemblies, classes, and recess. For example, if a student is mistreating a classmate, a teacher or principal might ask the student, "Are you living our vision here? Is your action a 'loving' one if you just slapped someone in the face?"

The physical education teacher explained that the school's success committees were derived from the mission and vision statement. The success committees focus on literacy, harmony, and wellness. In alignment with the statements, all three committees facilitate "learning." The literacy committee monitors academic successes. Students are "living, loving, and laughing" through the wellness committee that promotes good health and active living. The school success team promotes harmony by ensuring that students show appreciation and respect for different cultures.

In addition to the high standards set for students as learners, there are also high standards placed on conduct and character—social responsibility, citizenry, and simple good manners. Students learn to be good to themselves and others. This is also a school at which teachers both inside and outside the school report they want to work. Consider the workplace environment these teachers enjoy. There is reduced incidence of disruption and discontent. Students enjoy being at school and appreciate what they learn. Students and teachers enjoy each other's company and trust and respect each other. Teachers are supported in their efforts to expand and enrich programs by linking learning to their mission statement. This adds clarity and coherence to their teaching and learning initiatives and goals. This health-promoting school is a place where gaps are narrowed between knowing and doing, aspiration and achievement, and hope and happening.

Case Study

By Doug Gleddie

Your principal has asked you to be the healthy school community lead for Less-Than-Healthy K-9 School (LTH K-9). At the beginning of the year, therefore, you took a student leadership team (two Grade 5 and two Grade 6 students) to a Healthy Active School Symposium hosted by Ever Active Schools. You learned a lot, the students are pumped, and you have decided to begin transforming your school into a health-promoting one! You and your student leaders have made presentations to both the staff and the parent council. At both meetings, the response was ... underwhelming.

Unfortunately, you were told, in no uncertain terms, that, "We just don't have the time or resources for health promotion at LTH K-9. After all, we are a school, not a health centre!" You and your students, however, remain undaunted and prepared for change. A memorable question you once heard a keynote speaker ask keeps running through your head: "When will we use what we know, to change what we do?" You and your students get to work.

1. Why might parents and staff feel unenthusiastic about efforts to create a health-promoting school? Discuss the pressures and constraints that might act as barriers.
2. Using some of the WHO guidelines for HPS, how might you begin changing minds (and hearts and bodies) at LTH K-9?
3. Consider the JCSH Four Pillars model. Which pillar might be an effective place to start change? Why that pillar? Why that change?
4. How would you shift health promotion at this school from being something only you and four students are championing to "the way LTH K-9 does business"?

It's Your Turn

1 Where do you think your school is in the HPS process? Your district? Your province?

2 Identify and describe the role of external and internal influences in the development of health promotion in your school community.

3 What local and provincial supports are available to your school?

4 Check out the Healthy School Planner on the JCSH website and initiate a process evaluation at your school. Start with yourself—and build from there!

✓ Action Checklist

Individual	Suggested Follow-up
Pre-service Teacher	❑ Consider the evidence for HPS practice or process in your practicum school and ask if there might be a role for you. ❑ Share with peers and mentors suggestions for resources for HPS that you learned about in your teacher education classes. ❑ "Buddy up" with other pre-service teachers to discuss how to apply HPS concepts in each of your school communities.
Health and Physical Education Teacher	❑ Consider how you can extend your leadership from H&PE in order to connect to a broader HPS perspective. ❑ Seek out others from outside your area with whom to collaborate on this school-wide focus. ❑ Be sure to link health and physical education-related events and curriculum to HPS pillars and guidelines.
Administrator	❑ Educate parents and staff on the rationale for HPS. ❑ Inquire about district and provincial policies for healthy schools and make strides to implement or create policies as needed. ❑ Support staff, students, and parents, guardians to move HPS beyond events and presentations and into your school community.
Parent / Guardian	❑ Ask administration and teachers how they are incorporating student health and healthy school community practice in their daily decisions. ❑ Volunteer to serve on a healthy school committee. ❑ Support your child's healthy school with healthy practices at home and in the community.
Health Promotion Coordinator	❑ Connect with the health and physical education leader in the school as a place to start. ❑ Become familiar with school, district, and provincial policies for HPS. ❑ Realizing that school staff have a lot on their plate, ask how you can help and provide support to make things easier. ❑ Make a concerted effort to understand the education setting and vocabulary—you are in "their" world so it is up to you to adapt!

Chapter 2 Summary

The concept of the health-promoting school continues to evolve. Under the Comprehensive School Health framework, schools are uniquely positioned to serve as a catalyst and support mechanism for communities. Not only can schools directly affect the health and well-being of their students, but they can both directly and indirectly affect the health and well-being of the wider community. By extending health beyond the classroom as a strictly curricular subject to a mindset that advocates for a healthy physical environment, supportive social environments, and community partnerships, healthy schools can help instill the knowledge, skills, and attitudes needed for communities to make long-lasting, healthy choices.

Health promotion works best when the entire school is involved. A single classroom is an important start, but health promotion should be contagious, spreading throughout the school community. Health promotion, as we try to show throughout this book, provides a perspective from which to think about how to make life good: the relationships that make life good, the contributions that are part of a good life, and the goods in life that enable us to be happy.

Questions for Reflection

1 What partner organizations and individuals could be involved in planning and carrying out a healthy schools program within a CSH framework? How can they be identified and recruited?

2 What steps are involved in deciding which healthy school initiatives to pursue? In what ways is this process best initiated?

3 What resources are required to ensure successful implementation of HPS initiatives?

4 What role should the principal play in a health-promoting school?

5 How might the school community council be involved in a health-promoting school?

6 In what ways can students be given opportunities for meaningful involvement and leadership roles in school health promotion?

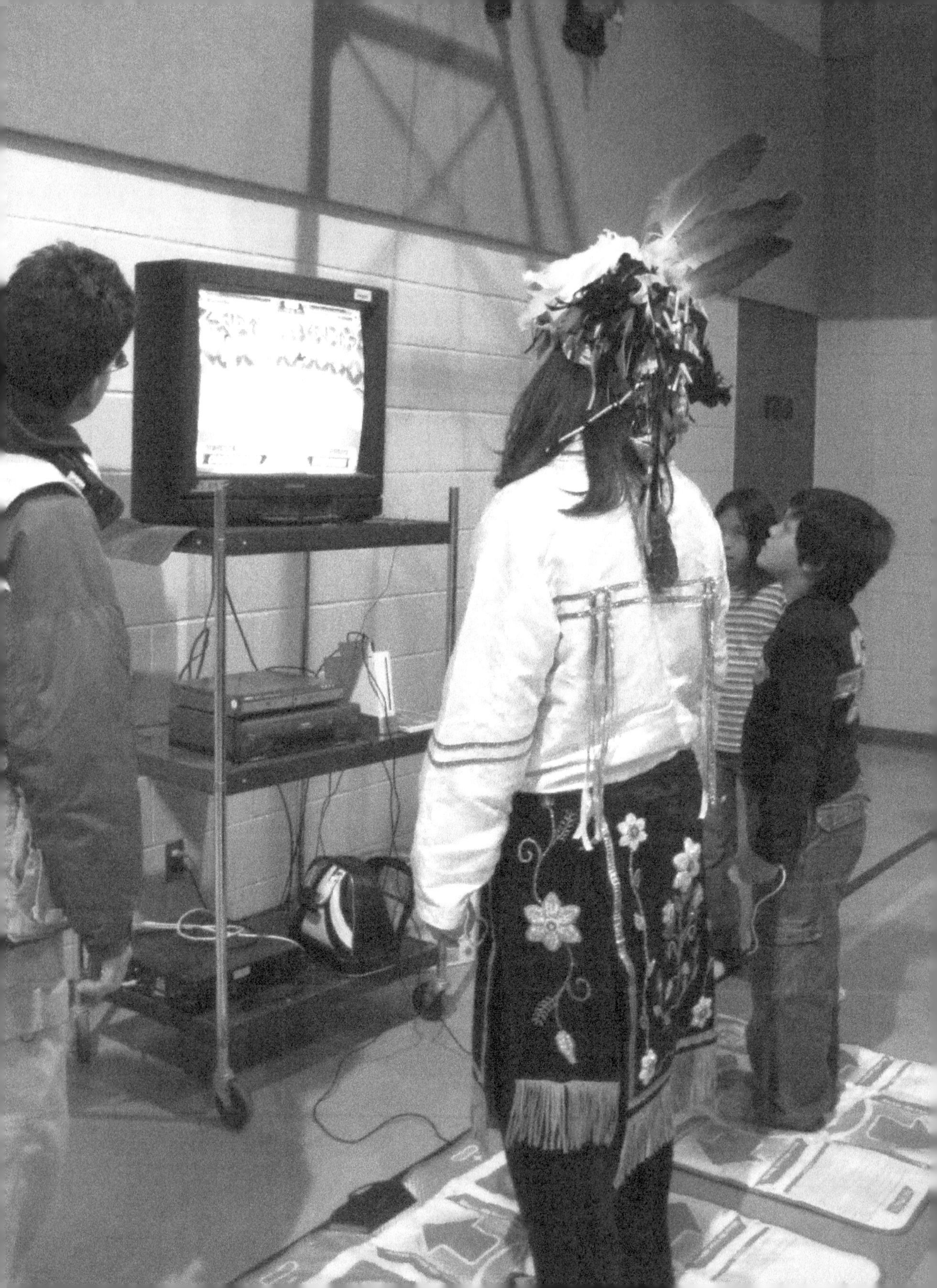

3

Instruction and Learning

The important role of teachers

Education is at the heart of health-promoting schools. High-quality instruction and programs are the foundation of the comprehensive school health model. The study of health should help students understand more fully about what matters to them—what values, passions, and beliefs underlie their decisions and actions. Expressions of health reflect personal goals, values, and hopes. Through explorations of health, educators contribute to students' formation of identity and personhood. Much is gained through health education, but most important may be the overall development of a person who is emotionally intelligent and aware of oneself and others.

Great teachers help students make choices that benefit not only them, but others around them as well. Great teachers inspire students to reach higher, value learning, get excited about content, and see themselves as contributors to the process of learning. Conversely, poor teachers make students feel left out, helpless, incompetent, and discouraged. Students who are continually exposed to autocratic teaching and rigid discipline by inadequately prepared teachers often display antisocial behaviour that negatively affects their health (Salas, 1997). Teacher excellence is distinguished in both the method and the manner by which teachers, students, and content interact.

Biology gives you a brain. Life turns it into a mind.

— Deffrey Eugenides, 2002, p.419.

Excellent teachers create ways to engage students such that more students learn more. Excellent teaching makes content more accessible through methods of instruction that:

- help students build knowledge instead of simply accumulating facts and information
- pose problems to be examined, rather than simply ask questions for which the teacher has ready-made answers
- facilitate further inquiry and exploration among students through discussion, experimentation, role playing, and abstract and imaginative thinking
- encourage students to demonstrate their understanding using multiple methods of knowledge presentation, including visual arts, music, drama, and poetry
- raise awareness of the ways in which students think and reason about issues
- integrate subject-area knowledge and skills with assessment and classroom management strategies
- encourage students to reason ethically, that is, by linking knowledge to helping others, responsible living, and citizenry

Excellence in teaching generates the following benefits:

- promotes inclusion by adopting a wide array of teaching methods, strategies, and lesson designs to ensure that all students enjoy rich and varied opportunities to learn
- promotes democracy by engaging students in learning activities and challenges whereby students apply what they are learning to real-life situations and to making a difference in the world
- promotes empowerment by teaching students about the learning process so they can self-regulate, manage their responsibilities, and be creative about their grasp and use of knowledge
- further promotes empowerment by providing students with a deep orientation to subject matter
- gives students chances to relate knowing to doing things better and doing better things
- prepares young people to relate learning to care for self and others

> ***Research has clearly shown that a good teacher is the single most important factor affecting student learning, more important than standards, class size or money*** —Geringer, 2003, p. 375

Because of excellence in teaching, students assume greater responsibility for attaining learning outcomes. Consequently, they come to own the knowledge, using it to open their minds and eyes to the perception of new meanings and to explore their presence in the world more deeply. Excellence in teaching is one of the best ways to ensure that the benefits of schooling reach as many children and youth as possible in ways that inspire them to be lifelong, confident, and capable learners.

Excellence in teaching is, therefore, at the heart of a nation's concerns about democracy and its capacity for sustainable and responsible growth.

> ***At its best, school can be about how to make a life, which is quite different from how to make a living.***—Postman, 1996

Among goals shared by teachers around the world, doing our best for our students is a top priority. Optimizing students' exposure to the most progressive and engaging methods of instruction should help ensure that all students will have the best chances to learn.

The purpose of this chapter is to demonstrate the critical importance of excellence in instruction and learning within a health-promoting school. The chapter discusses issues pertaining to the development of health literacy, the integration of health into other subject areas, and effective pedagogical strategies that can deliver quality instruction.

Learning about Health through Instruction

What are bruises? How does a cut heal? What is a healthy food? Why do our eyes water? Why do people sweat? Students have fascinating questions about growing up, how their bodies work, and how to take care of themselves. These concerns intensify as they become more conscious of messages (especially contradictory messages) that they receive at home, from friends, and from various forms of media. For example, a common exercise myth is that the more you sweat, the more fat you burn. This myth has led some people to believe that exercise while wearing a garbage bag will cause weight loss. Some companies looking to profit from this myth went as far as to sell products that increased sweating by counteracting the body's natural cooling mechanism.

In the classroom, teachers can encourage students to question prevailing and trending ideas as a way to promote critical, creative, and divergent thinking. The study of health as an invitation to wonder more deeply about self, others, and events in the world should give educators an opportunity to promote the skills of inquiry, observation, analysis, questioning, and research. Education with health in mind puts personal lives, emotions, circumstances, and values at the centre of knowledge making, decision making, and the action-planning process.

The Role of Health Education and Integrated School Health

It is estimated that well over 90% of the world's young people attend primary education (United Nations, 2015). Schools therefore offer one of the best opportunities to reach a majority of children and youth and equip them with the skills they need to lead healthy and active lives. A school is the one place in our society where every person should have equal and equitable access to learning opportunities that have a positive impact on their health.

Across Canada, however, health education is often marginalized. Despite the inclusion of many critical health topics—such as social relationships; safety; self-esteem; personal wellness; use, misuse, and abuse of substances; mental health; media literacy; and sexual health—a very small percentage of teaching time is devoted to health education in schools (Wright, 2006). The result is that the health curriculum is often overshadowed and hence under-delivered due to a severe lack of time and an insufficient number of health-education specialists in schools.

However, health concepts should not be limited strictly to the health-education curricula. They can be integrated into other subject areas as well. Integration means to make whole or complete; but complete does not mean finished or static. Rather, the completeness that integration affords is through opportunities to explore topics from multiple perspectives. This extends and makes prominent the variety, depth, and interrelationships that feed into diverse fields of study. Critics of integration complain that it weakens the curriculum and distracts students from paying attention to the primary elements of subject-matter study. They would argue, for example, that if you are studying mathematics, you should stick to mathematics.

Consider, however, how integration could enliven students' learning about a topic such as why angles matter. A student teacher was asked why she was teaching her Grade 5 class about the different kinds of angles. She replied that learning about angles is an explicit expectation in the math program. When asked why it is important for students to know about angles, she replied, "Because it's on the test. If I had more time I could find out how we use angles, but for now I just use the textbook." But imagine how richer the instruction would be if it included a real-world anecdote, such as the following, that features Canadian astronaut Chris Hadfield. He tells a story about something wondrous that happened in space. As he looked out the window of his spacecraft, Hadfield saw a beam of light reaching from Earth into space. He contacted mission control to inquire about the source of the beam of light. Curious, the team searched for an answer and then reported to Hadfield: "Chris, you'll never believe it. It's dawn in the Egyptian desert and the morning light is reflecting off the face of the pyramids and shining into space." Is it possible that the pyramids were constructed to do more than bury dead kings? Perhaps the position of the pyramids and the angles at which their walls were constructed were intended to do something quite extraordinary during ancient times, such as connecting with the gods. Linking subject-area topics that might otherwise seem dry to intriguing real-life mysteries and phenomena can serve to hook and sustain students' attention and their need to satisfy their boundless curiosity.

Done properly, integration enriches study within a curriculum area by broadening students' understanding of a topic and facilitating multiple dimensions of understanding. Rather than diminish the integrity of the subject matter, integration can amplify and diversify it. The lustre and quality of each stone in a jar of precious gems is enhanced by proximity to the others. Similarly, the study of health as an integral part of other areas of study such as mathematics, language arts, music, and dance adds context and personal meaning to learning, thereby enriching and enlivening academic study.

Connecting learning to life is at the heart of education. Great teachers bring concepts to life in ways that make learning relevant and allow students to experience learning's true importance. For example, learning about respect is not simply a means to avoid a trip to the principal's office. When respect is taught through a health lens, students begin to realize and experience for themselves that respect has much broader implications for one's self, others, and the environment. Respect for the environment, for example, can inspire actions to make the air we breathe cleaner or the communities in which we live safer and more conducive to outdoor activities.

Health as it is presented here is a way of integrating various areas of study so that different perspectives coalesce. Health topics afford opportunities to triangulate three critical dimensions of education:

- the acquisition of background knowledge
- the ability to apply, relate, and transfer knowledge to the development of skills that serve to build action competence (the ability to appropriately use what we know)
- the notion that learning to know and do is part of a process of becoming a better person

Inquiry into health topics and issues prompts the learner to go beyond "know" and "do" to examine the question: "What is it about this topic that matters to me/us in terms of making a good life for self and others?" To use an analogy: If we are planting trees, what is the forest we are creating?

Integrative approaches to health bring several different communities together: communities of scholarship, communities of decision makers, and communities of service. Integrative approaches promote deeper understanding of health. For example, sexual health can be explored from perspectives outside health studies, including culture, religion, sociology, and anthropology. Sexual health education studied exclusively from a single perspective, such as biomedical content—how the body works, disease prevention, and contraception—limits opportunities for students to develop comprehensive and meaningful understanding of issues and questions such as: When is the right time to have sex? What is love? Why can't we talk about pleasure and desire when we study sexual health? What role should parents and guardians play in education related to sexual health?

The key emphasis here is that education about health needs to exceed the boundaries of single subject-area study. Herein lies the significance of interdisciplinary study. Each discipline, and indeed the different strands within the health curriculum itself, afford learners opportunities to study topics from different vantage points. For example, why are certain groups of women more likely to become pregnant at an early age than others? Why are most contraception devices designed for women rather than for men? What factors influence birth rates in countries around the world? The unique perspectives of different disciplines give students a deeper understanding of the subjects themselves—what forms of knowledge are valued, how knowledge within this area of study is generated and communicated, and how knowledge relates to decision making.

Consider the different ways in which the heart can be studied from a physical health perspective: how the heart functions, the effects of physical activity on cardiac health, the relationship between heart health and smoking, and so forth. But when we think about the heart beyond the health curriculum, we open up a host of other opportunities for learning and discussion: What do we mean when we encourage someone to "take heart," to "play with heart," or to "have a heart"? What does it mean to "break someone's heart," to "die of a broken heart," or to extend to someone "heart-felt thanks"?

The study of health as an integral part of academic study is important because it humanizes subject-area content. Consider this situation involving a class in a neighbourhood challenged by high unemployment, poor housing, family discord, and violence. The class, which the teacher referred to as the "snake pit," consisted entirely of young males aged 16 or 17. The health topic the students were supposed to be studying was stress. The first thing they were assigned to do was to copy Hans Selye's definition of stress from the chalkboard. A few made an attempt to copy the words written on the board, but most were disengaged and spent most of the period shuffling papers, trying to find a notebook, or looking for a pencil or pen to complete the task.

What if the teacher had asked the students to talk about the stress they face daily? What if the students' real-life experiences were the curriculum of study? Ignoring what the students already know devalues their contribution to the learning process. In this example, forcing students to memorize a definition that meant nothing to them was ineffective and irrelevant—and demeaning.

What if a conversation with these young men revealed that the major stresses in their lives had to do with a sense of hopelessness? ("I'm never going to finish school and get a decent job. What have I got to lose by doing drugs?") How much more influential would instruction be if the real issues in these students' lives were valued? How much more inviting would a school be if concerted efforts were made to understand and reflect the realities of students' lives in the way in which students were taught?

Under these conditions, health can become a way of studying, taking note of, and shaping events in the world. For students, embedding health in content and vice versa (relating academic study to current health concerns) can become a way to connect content, culture, and context. This allows student to build a bridge between academics and their own life pursuits. By integrating health with other subjects, teachers can:

- enliven the content
- confront the realities of contemporary society
- present opportunities to explore issues from diverse perspectives
- participate in efforts to create a just society
- experience and promote contribution through service

SUCCESS STORY

Hope Blooms

By Jane McNulty

In 2008, the city of Halifax turned over a piece of abandoned land that was full of garbage and weeds to a fledgling community start-up group calling themselves "Hope Blooms." Today, that piece of land has been transformed into a flourishing hub of meaningful teaching and learning experiences that include a community garden, a solar-powered greenhouse, a commercial kitchen, and a social enterprise run by at-risk youth whose efforts directly impact the social determinants of health in their communities.

Hope Blooms was founded by Jessie Jollymore, a community dietitian working in Halifax's North End inner-city neighbourhood. Concerned about food security issues, poverty, and chronic illness, Jessie saw that simply telling people about the importance of a healthy diet was not helpful or effective. When people cannot afford to buy healthy food, they are left feeling helpless and hopeless. So, Jessie decided to rally young members of the community to create a non-profit community vegetable garden. Despite warnings that the garden would be vandalized, it is thriving today. More than 50 youth and their families are changing their neighbourhood for the better by demonstrating that "when you change the way you look at things, the things you look at change."

The young people who roll up their sleeves to become part of Hope Blooms acquire many practical skills through hands-on learning. They learn how to grow food, produce and market their own healthy products such as organic herbal salad dressings, develop and maintain a small social enterprise, and give back to their community. They not only *participate* in this community-based model—they *lead* it and *shape* it to needs of their families and of the wider community as well. Their efforts have replaced the neighbourhood's patterns of dependency and isolation with the power of ownership and self-determination.

The learning has extended well beyond the city of Halifax and even the province of Nova Scotia. Herbs from the community garden are processed into organic salad dressings that are sold to finance a student scholarship fund and community nutrition projects. In 2013, a group of young entrepreneurs representing Hope Blooms were able to expand their salad dressing business and build a greenhouse after travelling to Toronto and landing a $40,000 investment from the CBC reality show "Dragons' Den." The greenhouse sits next to the garden and has become a teaching and learning resource for the whole community. It has allowed Hope Blooms to double its salad dressing production to more than 15,000 bottles a year!

Instead of using electricity from the grid to heat the greenhouse, some of the 50 students in Hope Blooms brainstormed energy alternatives with architects who donated time to the project. They figured out how to use energy from garden compost and organic materials such as coffee grounds and hops. The waste goes into compost bins outside the greenhouse and pipes convey the energy generated by the compost under and up through the floor of the greenhouse to heat it.

In May 2017, Hope Blooms began expanding their garden plot on Brunswick Street to make room for 15 Syrian families in the neighbourhood and to lend their kitchen out to another non-profit, Piece of the East, that up-cycles food for people in need.

The Hope Blooms model is strong because it is built upon a foundation of community relationships. With a focus on collaborative and sustainable practices, its programs provide a platform that emphasizes community assets, not liabilities, in meaningfully addressing issues such as food insecurity, social exclusion, and poor health. A student-led initiative built on trust, inclusivity, and the recognition that everyone has something to offer and that every voice is heard and respected has created a space where youth feel equal, valued, and empowered to take control over their futures.

As aptly stated on the Hope Blooms website: "For youth today, there are few places where they feel they have control over anything or where they can be themselves without judgement. Hope Blooms youth are empowered to take control and actively steer the direction the program takes. In doing so, they take ownership over their contributions and are able to experience the true freedoms of their own efforts. Through hosting monthly community suppers for upwards of 40 people, teaching other youth, parents, and neighbours how to grow food, preparing organic soups for seniors, or donating portions of the herb dressing proceeds to supporting other community building efforts, these youth are learning and teaching others that the path to self-actualization is also a path to generosity." ■

Health Literacy

The overall goal of health education and integrated school health is the development of health literacy. Freire and Macedo (1987) refer to literacy as the ability to "not only read the word but to also read the world." In other words, it is not only about the knowledge that we collect; rather, it is about how we use that knowledge to make our world a better place in which to live. Literacy creates a deeper and broader understanding of issues within and across subject areas. It helps to stimulate further inquiry and ideas by making connections to real-life issues. If we consider the kind of thinking that is associated with being a "literate" person, the idea of literacy becomes clearer.

The Public Health Agency of Canada defines health literacy as "the ability to access, comprehend, evaluate and communicate information as a way to promote, maintain and improve health in a variety of settings across the life-course."[1] In 1994, the Joint Committee on National Health Education Standards in the United States presented health literacy as the life skills of health promotion. Education for health literacy consists of four key components: a) critical thinking and problem solving skills, b) responsible and productive citizenship, c) self-directed learning; and, d) effective communication.

- Critical thinking. Young people who are critical thinkers can examine personal, national, and international health problems and then formulate ideas as to how these problems might be solved. They gather and assess information from a variety of sources before making health-related decisions. They approach health promotion via creative thinking processes and make informed decisions.
- Responsible citizenship. Young people who are responsible and productive citizens feel obligated to keep their community healthy, safe, and secure. They believe that all citizens deserve a high quality of life, and they realize that their behaviour affects the quality of life for others. Thus, they work collaboratively with others, maintaining and improving health for all citizens.
- Self-directed learning. Young people who are self-directed learners understand that information about healthy lifestyles and health prevention will change as research advances. During their lifetime, they will be advocates for their own health, continually gathering new information that will aid in making healthy choices. With advanced skills in literacy, numeracy, and critical thinking, self-directed learners are also able to follow instructions from others, and have developed the interpersonal skills to do so. Having internalized this learning process, self-directed learners use it to progress toward a high level of wellness as they grow and mature.
- Effective communication. Young people who are effective communicators can express ideas and convey their knowledge through multiple channels—orally, in writing, artistically, graphically, and through technological media. They demonstrate empathy and respect for others, and encourage others to express

1 Public Health Agency of Canada. Available at: https://www.canada.ca/en/public-health/services/chronic-diseases/health-literacy.html.

themselves. They also listen carefully and respond when others speak. Finally, they are advocates for positions, policies, and programs that promote healthy lifestyles.

Nutbeam's (2000) discussion of health literacy focuses on three aspects designed to:

- prepare students to obtain relevant health information: functional literacy
- relate knowledge of health and interpersonal skills to personal/social situations: interactive literacy
- reflect on the underlying issues and environmental factors (e.g., racial and ethnic concerns, economic and social status) and political and cultural factors that impact opportunities to be healthy: critical literacy

To achieve **functional literacy,** educators can teach reading strategies that enable students to make connections to a variety of health texts: articles, blogs, magazines, videos, and advertisements that contain messages about health and the roles people play in achieving good health. Many weight-loss commercials, for example, make claims that sound "too good to be true." Teachers committed to health promotion encourage students to question the logic behind unrealistic health claims and to look to health professionals who are not "selling" anything for information and advice.

Other reading strategies include the ability to interpret procedural or technical information such as that found on prescriptions and medication labels. What exactly does one pill three times a day mean? Should you take one pill at 8-hour intervals, or can you take all three pills at once?

Interactive literacy focuses on the interactions between people, because often decisions about health are closely linked to our relationships. If your friends are involved in physical-activity pursuits, you are likely to join them. Similarly, if your friends smoke, you are more likely to smoke. Students need to examine the reasons why people value friendships, but also consider their need to become independent persons. Students developing interactive literacy will develop a number of communication skills (listening, assertiveness, and critical thinking) as well as a higher degree of emotional intelligence (empathy, sincerity, and kindness). Knowing where others are coming from, and then deciding where to stand in relation to them is part of becoming a literate person.

Role playing is often a useful way to explore feelings and language. It is also a way to rehearse situations and re-write scripts that might occur later in life. Puppetry, dance, tableaux, videos, and poster presentations can also be used to highlight the importance of being true to yourself and your values, hopes, and dreams.

Critical literacy involves becoming a more discerning consumer of information and products. Critically literate students can:

- identify credible print sources and web sites related to a current health issue
- analyze and present data from individuals who are not members of their health class

- identify critical questions related to an issue; for example, if nutrition is so important, why do we sometimes sell junk food as part of fundraising initiatives at schools? If physical activity is such an important part of our growth and development, why do we only have physical education twice a week for 30 minutes? How can developing nations make profits selling illegal drugs when they don't have drugs for HIV infection?
- synthesize information related to an issue and present a health issues information sheet
- verbally communicate important aspects of an issue to other students: for example, who gets more air time in the media related to achievements in sport—men or women; persons with disabilities or persons without disabilities? (From Birch, 2000, p. 69)

Approaches that centre on the development of critical-thinking skills feature a process whereby students start by addressing a problem or scenario. It often begins with a question or statement presented by the teacher. It may also occur unexpectedly in the classroom, on the playground, or from a story reported in the news. For example, "Of what value are tattoos?" From this question a web of ideas and other questions flow: For how long has tattooing been around? How is a tattoo inscribed? For what purposes have tattoos been used on people and on animals? What are the health risks of getting a tattoo? Before judgments about tattooing can be made, students must first build a knowledge base—get the facts, the story, and the details. To do so, they may need to develop specialized tools for learning, such as interviewing techniques, Internet search strategies, library search methods, art analysis, and so on. Then they must develop some criteria about choices related to tattooing. Finally, they can present their findings and conclusions in the form of well-constructed arguments and summaries.

Effective Pedagogy

Fundamental to the notion of instruction is understanding that learning and health are developmental. In other words, our sense of health progresses as knowledge and experience accrue. Concepts learned as a child develop into more sophisticated intellectual structures by the time we reach adulthood. However, advancement does not occur without the benefit of critical reflection. Immature interpretations may linger into adulthood unless they are transformed by more advanced ways of thinking. A teacher working with Grade 2 children studying the four food groups asked them to sort dozens of pictures of food commonly found in their lives—everything from ice cream and French fries to carrots. The teacher allowed the students to create food categories rather than simply adopt the ones taught in class. The food groups one group chose were: foods your parents make you eat, junk food, snacks, and treats. Interestingly, treats were often also found in the junk food category. Most of us "live by" food categories that do not necessarily fall into the categories that nutritionists prefer. We have, for example, comfort food, party food, knapsack food, microwave food, camping food, and so on.

Knowing is not enough. Unlike most other areas of the curriculum, health invites students to consider information worth knowing in relation to factors that impact real life. For instance, students of health are presented with information about the hazards of smoking, the reasons people smoke, the nature of addiction, and so on. Additionally, students explore environmental factors that influence the use of tobacco products, such as the fact that tobacco is a legal product for adults, sold in thousands of stores. Strategies to cope with peer pressure and stress are also a significant part of the content needed to promote the health behaviours associated with smoke-free living.

Contrast the need to examine social and economic barriers to good health with the way students are taught to read or use a computer. Imagine helping to inspire students to read more or to resist pressure from friends to play a particularly violent video game. Yet that is exactly how educators must socialize and personalize content when it is related to achieving desired health outcomes. Integrating health with academic study enables students to look at the developmental nature of knowledge and then relate knowledge to daily living. Reading with health in mind invites consideration of the social, economic, and emotional factors that impact reading: Do you have trouble concentrating when you read? Do you wish you could read more but just can't find the time? How do you cope with these feelings and situations?

Engaging Students in the Learning Process

Health education entails acting on beliefs and convictions. It should prepare students to engage in the process of change and as such expose students to roles of agency and responsible leadership. "The importance of process is yet another discovery. Goals and end points matter less. Learning is more urgent than storing information. Caring is better than keeping. Means are ends. The journey is the destination. When life becomes a process, the old distinctions between winning and losing, success and failure, fade away. Everything, even a negative outcome, has the potential to teach us and to further our quest." (Ferguson, 1980, p.101)

One of the fundamental outcomes of a good education is that students end up knowing more about how learning occurs (how the brain processes sensory input; how knowledge and skills are acquired, maintained, and used as part of daily living). Consider the following example. At one secondary school, a teacher worked with a group of students to redefine not just food choices but a school cafeteria's ideal role as part of the overall school and learning experience. They changed the name of the cafeteria to the Screaming Avocado Café, painted the walls to look more like a teen café than an army barracks, and played music that students wanted to hear. They also contacted local chefs and an organic farmer to work with students to develop new recipes that eventually became part of the cafeteria menu. Students interested in the food and beverage industry worked with staff to help with food preparation, table service, and clean-up duties. These skills proved to be transferable to employment opportunities and built interest in the culinary arts as a vocation gained through post-graduate and apprenticeship study. This secondary school has also started an organic garden and is now producing its own vegetables.

The relationship between learning and emotion should also be a prominent part of classroom life. How might students benefit from examining the effects of loneliness, teasing, or apathy about learning on one's mental health? Conversely, how is learning influenced by feelings of self-worth and optimism, and acts of empathy, kindness, and helpfulness toward others? More specifically, students might learn the importance of thinking about their talents and imaginations as tools that enable them to think positively and strategically about how to handle everyday problems. Learning with health in mind might foster opportunities to support what Seligman (1998) termed *learned optimism* (that is, the belief that within each of us are the resources, ideas and insights, and ability to work together that are needed to overcome adversity and challenges). Goleman (1995) uses the term *emotional intelligence* to describe the importance of having a strong expectation that, in general, things will turn out all right in life, despite setbacks and frustrations. Optimism is an attitude that buffers people against falling into apathy, hopelessness, or depression in the face of tough challenges.

Canadian-born Jean Vanier founded L'Arche in 1964 to create open, inclusive, and compassionate communities that welcome and support people with intellectual disabilities. Vanier maintains that there is a universal order to life that we must learn to recognize and harness to ensure we achieve our human potential and live with dignity. Knowing, linked intimately to the way people live their lives, enables students to be able to appreciate that knowledge is constructed in relation to culture, community, and context. Therefore, knowing is value-laden, temporal, and subjective. Accordingly, for a subject to be learned well, students must master the background thinking associated with that subject. Students encouraged to think about content as a form of cultural expression are in a better position to reason, analyze, apply, and transfer knowing to different situations, solve problems, anticipate consequences, detect errors, and create alternative plans for action.

Consider, for example, how differently health is addressed in Western cultures compared to Indigenous cultures. In Western cultures, health is predominantly understood and organized in relation to what is happening inside the body—(micro) biologically and biochemically. Health is managed medicinally through the administration of pharmaceutical and surgical interventions that seek to monitor, regulate, or alter cellular activity. A check-up entails extraction of body fluids, and blood pressure and temperature readings to produce numerical data that are cross-referenced with population norms. In contrast, Indigenous worldviews define health in terms of a person's relationships with the natural world. Central to these worldviews is harmony with the Earth—plants, animals, soil, sun, and water. Thus, a health check-up might involve more personal and reflective approaches, such as those practised by the Haida Indians: hiking in the mountains, bathing in cool spring waters at dawn, and meditating on one's place and purpose on Earth.

Case Study

By Amanda Stanec

Elliott is preparing for next year's teaching assignment that includes four sections of English and one section of health education. He is thrilled because it is the first time he has been assigned to teach health and it is a subject that he values both personally and professionally.

Committed to living a healthy life, Elliott is often teased jovially by his co-workers for bringing healthy lunches and staying focused on his jogging goals. In his B.Ed. program, Elliott majored in physical education, with English as his second teachable subject. During pre-service training two years ago, Elliott completed a course in health education instructional methods. It left a positive and life-changing impression on him.

Looking at healthy living from a comprehensive and holistic perspective, Elliott now wonders why health is mostly viewed as an add-on rather than a core subject at the middle school where he teaches. Elliott is concerned that his school is not doing enough to prepare students to make independent decisions that positively impact their health, as well as the health of those around them. He wants to work to normalize quality health education within the school and in the surrounding community.

Elliott recently saw one of his administrators at a community function. The administrator commented that while she is happy that Elliott is excited to teach health, he needs to understand that school and district rankings rely heavily on high English scores. Elliott commented that students are unlikely to perform their best in any content area if they are not learning about making healthy choices to benefit themselves and others. However, the administrator made it very clear that she expected Elliott to model excellence in instruction in English first and to help students performing below expectations to improve to grade level and higher. Then, she told Elliott that she looked forward to hearing about his professional goals at the back-to-school goal-setting meeting that they would have early in the school year.

Elliott left the function feeling as though someone had let the wind out of his sails. How antiquated could someone be? Why, he wondered, do decision makers in education continue to ignore the science around health and learning? However, those feelings did not linger very long. Elliott became determined to promote health learning strategies that would let him support his students the way he knew best. He immediately went home and began to think about solutions to the challenges that had presented themselves that evening.

1 Put yourself in Elliott's shoes. What personal strengths (such as leadership and organizational skills, work experience) would you bring to help navigate these challenges?
2 If you were Elliott, what goals would you establish for your back-to-school goal-setting meeting with the administrator? Is a strategy needed to present these goals in such a way that the administrator will support them? If so, what strategy do you suggest?
3 What forms of evidence would you bring to the table that demonstrate the efficacy of quality health education? How would you share this evidence with your administrator? How would you share this evidence with other staff members? With parents and guardians?

It's Your Turn

1 Develop short-term and long-term goals, as well as performance measures to track progress, in order to apply content from this chapter to your current setting.

2 Create an assessment strategy to determine the effectiveness of the goals in question 1.

✓ Action Checklist

Individual	Suggested Follow-up
Pre-service Teacher	❑ During practicum placements, seek out resources or units that focus on integrated learning—health should be the secondary content taught in these instances. ❑ Whenever possible, choose integrated learning strategies and planning as part of course assignments to gain competence and confidence in modelling excellent teaching through an integrated learning model. ❑ Take a chance and volunteer to teach health!
Health and Physical Education Teacher Health Education Teacher	❑ Collaborate closely with the teachers at your school and determine ways to integrate learning into one another's classes. ❑ Meet with experts from the health sector (e.g., public health nurse, paediatrician, health researcher) to ensure that topics are being covered in a comprehensive manner, and determine how to cover any topics that are not currently included. ❑ Educate colleagues on the importance of teaching health in all content areas and how they can do so by increasing meaningful connections for students. ❑ View yourself as a leader and a resource person for others and be approachable to others who may want to increase health-promoting norms in the school community. ❑ Educate teaching colleagues on how they can integrate skills-based health education into their content areas.
Administrator	❑ Provide professional development opportunities and resources for all teachers on how they can practise and model integrated teaching. ❑ Encourage and support teachers who teach subjects other than health to become motivated and committed to integrating health into those subject areas.
Parent / Guardian	❑ Ask school administrators how health is taught, how often health is taught, and if integrated teaching occurs to optimize health education. ❑ Ask health teachers to communicate what they are teaching so you can reinforce skills and concepts at home. ❑ Ask your child what they are learning about their health, and let teachers who are focusing on your child's health know that you value what they are doing.

Chapter 3 Summary

Teachers play a vital role in the healthy development of their students. They equip students with the knowledge, skills, and attitudes to make healthy choices—about what to eat, about being active, about compassion for others and the environment. Whatever the desired health outcome, teachers have the potential to instill in their students the life skills needed to recognize, communicate, and act on healthy choices.

Through health education, teachers can directly provide students with the knowledge and understanding, thinking, communication, and application skills needed to lead healthy active lives. Imagine the enthusiasm that students will have when they can learn about various cultures in social studies through cooperative games, or how learning sorting and matching skills in primary mathematics can come to life when students learn to group healthy foods together. When teachers and schools start to look through a health lens and make decisions using effective pedagogy, the result is a school community where all members have the opportunity to thrive and succeed.

Questions for Reflection

1 A teacher decided to take neighbourhood walks with her students to look for "homes" of insects, birds, squirrels, and other wildlife. Over time they developed a walk that told the story of the neighbourhood from many perspectives, such as history, architecture, gardens, and natural landscapes. What is healthy about a heritage walk?

2 A group of Grade 5 students learned about the formation of rocks millions of years ago. They learned that each stone has a story that helps reveal the history of Earth. After class, a student remarked she would never throw a stone away again because it is a kind of storybook. This student had been "struck" by the wonder of something as ordinary as a rock. What else might students wonder about when learning about rocks and geological formations?

3 Survey students about the occupations of their parents or guardians, other family members, or neighbours (being careful to respect students' privacy). With students, identify some ways in which workers in our communities perform different roles to help keep people healthy (e.g., a plumber installs pipes to deliver clean water; restaurant employees follow sanitary procedures to ensure that food is prepared safely; a police officer helps keep communities safe).

4 Survey students about their favourite physical activities and, if time permits, invite students to create a bulletin board display or post videos to the school website. Identify as well the different places where students can be physically active in their community.

5 What strategies or persuasive messaging might help to motivate teachers who teach subjects such as math or Language Arts to begin to integrate a health strand throughout their teaching if they are not already doing so?

6 Describe what you would consider to be an ideal team of health-promoting educators in terms of their goals, personal qualities, and teaching methods.

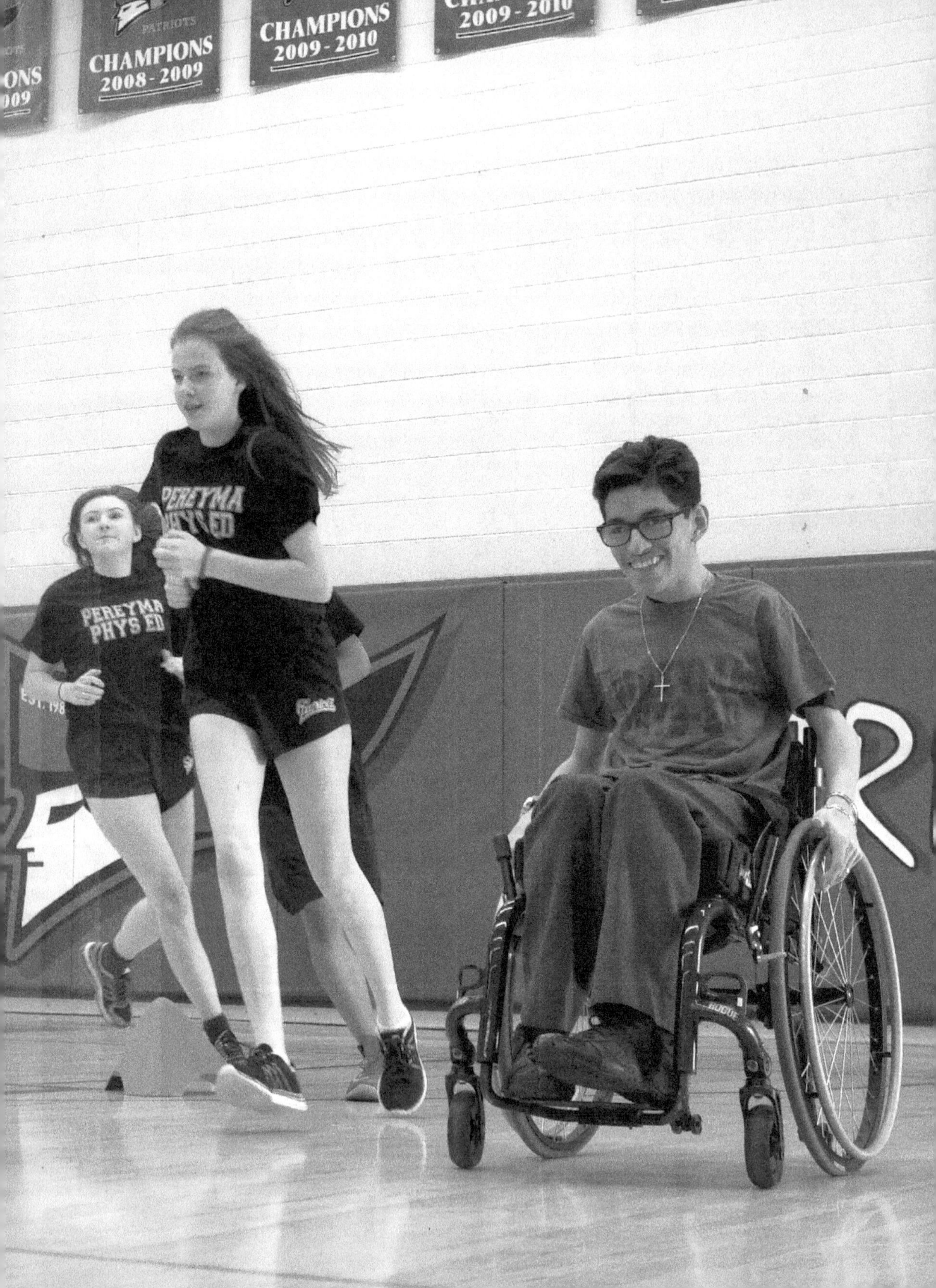
CHAMPIONS
2008 - 2009
CHAMPIONS
2009 - 2010
2009 - 2010
PEREYMA
PHYS ED

4

The Physical Environment and Health-Promoting Schools

Building community

Ideally, schools should not only look and feel like health-promoting schools—they should also offer students multiple opportunities to apply their knowledge of health in many different contexts. It is important that a school's messaging and culture encourage students to be physically active, choose healthy foods, and get sufficient sleep and rest. But if playground equipment is falling apart, if vending machines serve only high-sugar drinks, or if there are no bicycle racks for students to store their bikes safely, students will be less likely to make healthy, active choices.

Educators often work hard to shape a school into an oasis, a safe haven, or an inviting place for children to share a large and important part of their lives growing up and learning together. What is the role of the school's physical environment in creating such an inviting space? Playgrounds, the school structure itself, and landscaping not only help support a healthy learning environment, but also provide opportunities for students to apply their knowledge of health in creative and innovative ways. A growing body of research demonstrates that health is nurtured through school-ground naturalization, greening the school environment inside and outside, and collaboration among all members of the school community to make the school a place where learning is valued and reflected in many functional and aesthetically pleasing ways.

Anthropologist and primatologist Jane Goodall, who has devoted her life to the study of chimpanzees in their natural habitats, encourages everyone to do as she has for decades—marvel at the mystery and beauty of nature. A towering tree, grass gently swaying in the breeze, a newborn, or a bird soaring in the sky are evidence that we are part of something much greater than ourselves. The more opportunities we have to observe nature with wonder and curiosity—to see its majesty, power, gentleness, and forgiveness—the more nature can awaken within us a sense of hope and possibility. Here are some examples of initiatives that school communities have undertaken to enhance engagement with nature.

- Urban farms. More and more urban communities are developing plots of land to grow vegetables and flowers for communal use. As a community, people come together to plan, plant, and enjoy the results. Families learn more about and begin to care more for other community members. Children gain the experience of working in the soil, learning about plant life, and enjoying the fruits of their labour.
- Schools in Bloom. Entire school communities support the beautification of schoolyards through programs that teach about and help financially support plantings and schoolyard maintenance. Organic gardens, peace gardens, heritage gardens, and Shakespearean gardens can bring together the entire school population and landscape designers to collaborate on a Schools in Bloom initiative shared by schools throughout a district or province.
- Schoolyard makeovers. Capitalizing on the idea of a makeover can rally a school around a project aimed at making the schoolyard inviting, safe, and aesthetically pleasing. What organisms besides humans might visit these spaces—butterflies, insects, birds? What might attract these organisms to the schoolyard?

It is well documented that environmental improvement can lead to positive changes in behaviour patterns. Students involved in the planning and care of school improvement projects experience an increased sense of belonging and a sense of ownership. Aggression, vandalism, litter, and graffiti are all less likely and less tolerated in a school community where everyone cooperates to create and sustain an enjoyable environment (Ann Coffey, Green School Project, Ottawa, as cited in Raffan, 2000).

Physical Safety in the School Environment

This sometimes-overlooked aspect of a healthy school is crucial to students' well-being and development. Physical safety in school communities depends on specific rules and regulations (such as WHMIS standards), guidelines for physical activity (e.g., the Ontario Physical Education Safety Guidelines), policies for safe and healthy active transportation, field trip regulations, and more. Here are some broad categories that physical safety covers:

1 Safety guidelines for physical activity. Although these guidelines are superseded by site-specific school authority policies (established by local school boards and schools), they establish a minimum standard of care for students

and staff involved in a wide variety of physical activities organized by the school. Inter-school sports, intramurals, physical education, and off-site field trips are all covered by these guidelines. Also included are safety standards for equipment such as gymnastic mats and playground structures, as well as for gymnasiums, fitness rooms, and other facilities. Safety guidelines are evergreen documents—they are updated regularly to include new and emerging activities and to reflect occasional changes in workplace safety standards, for example.

2 Active transportation. One of the simplest ways to incorporate more physical activity into each school day is to support the use of active transport. Encouraging students to run, walk, wheel, or roll their way to school is a natural fit for a healthy school community. Safe Healthy Active People Everywhere (SHAPE) provides a variety of supports for those looking to improve active and safe modes of transportation. The organization publishes a manual that offers a wealth of information on:
   - traffic: a child's point of view
   - research about why active transport is important
   - tips for identifying and promoting safe routes to and from school
   - ideas for safe drop-off zones for students; specified distances at which bussed students will be dropped off and picked up
   - ways to establish safe walking areas around the school (such as attentiveness to ice or cracks in pavement); crossing guards at busy intersections
   - suggestions for securing bicycles, skateboards, and scooters while students are in school

   More information about how to promote active transportation appears later in this chapter.

3 The school campus. Most school authorities have policies and guidelines to cover a wide variety of safety procedures and features related to building security. Take the time to become familiar with policies and guidelines applicable to your school and district to be sure your students have an optimal environment in which to learn and play:
   - regulations and procedures related to school visitors (e.g., notices requesting that visitors report immediately to the main office upon entering the school)
   - lockdown procedures in the event of a threat of violence or an attack upon students and staff
   - policies related to possession of weapons and dangerous or illicit substances
   - vigilant playground/lunchroom/cafeteria supervision policies and procedures, including staff-to-student ratios
   - first-aid stations, defibrillating stations, and posted procedures for responding to emergencies such as CPR and dealing with concussions
   - fire safety: signs, drills, and procedures

- safe and adequate lighting, heating, air conditioning, and ventilation
- safe food-handling practices, safe food storage and temperatures, and safe food-handling certification and training
- safety for student leaders when cooking/preparing food for activities such as breakfast clubs and fundraisers
- policies and procedures for managing food allergies/sensitivities
- hand washing, use of hand sanitizers, and general hygiene (e.g., sneezing into the elbow)

Accessibility and Inclusion

Another important aspect of the physical environment is accessibility and inclusion. Many new schools are built using a concept known as universal design in education (UDE) for products and environments. According to the Center for Universal Design in Education at the University of Washington, the practice of "UDE goes beyond accessible design for people with disabilities to make all aspects of the educational experience more inclusive for students, parents, staff, instructors, administrators, and visitors with a great variety of characteristics. These characteristics include those related to gender, race and ethnicity, age, stature, disability, and learning style" (Burgstahler, 2015, p. 1).

The seven principles of universal design are:

1. Equitable use. The design is useful and marketable to people with diverse abilities. Career services example: Job postings in formats accessible to people with a broad range of abilities, disabilities, ages, and racial and ethnic backgrounds.
2. Flexibility in use. The design accommodates a wide range of individual preferences and abilities. Campus museum example: A design that allows a visitor to choose to read or listen to the description of the contents of display cases.
3. Simple and intuitive use. Use of the design is easy to understand, regardless of the user's experience, knowledge, language skills, or current concentration level. Assessment example: Testing in a predictable, straightforward manner.
4. Perceptible information. The design communicates necessary information effectively to the user, regardless of ambient conditions or the user's sensory abilities. Dormitory example: An emergency alarm system with visual, aural, and kinesthetic characteristics.
5. Tolerance for error. The design minimizes hazards and the adverse consequences of accidental or unintended actions. Instructional software example: A program that provides guidance when the student makes an inappropriate selection.

6 **Low physical effort.** The design can be used efficiently and comfortably and with a minimum of fatigue. Curriculum example: Software with on-screen control buttons that are large enough for students with limited fine-motor skills to select easily.

7 **Size and space for approach and use.** Appropriate size and space are provided for approach, reach, manipulation, and use regardless of the user's body size, posture, or mobility. Science lab example: An adjustable table and work area that can be used by students who are right- or left-handed and who have a wide range of physical characteristics and abilities.

To visualize what these principles of universal design might look like in a healthy school community, reflect on these questions:

- Are the school's physical spaces designed to enhance access for all students?
- Does the school offer a variety of facilities and equipment such that students of all ages, genders, developmental stages, and abilities can participate in games and sports and enjoy playground equipment and playing fields to every extent possible?
- What provisions are or could be made for students with special needs as well as for reluctant learners?
- What provisions are or could be made for students with complex needs?
- Do all students have opportunities for physical activity outside of curriculum time and access to appropriate resources: gymnasium, other large room suitable for physical activity (e.g., auditorium, cafeteria, or dance studio), outdoor facilities, and equipment such as balls, skipping ropes, playground equipment, skates, or snowshoes?
- Does the school's planning process include possible renovation or redesign of school spaces to increase accessibility? Can upgrades of existing school spaces incorporate accessibility features?
- What grants or funding opportunities are available to facilitate such upgrades?

Increasing Opportunities for Active Transportation

The title of the 2013 Report Card on Physical Activity for Children and Youth asks, "Are we driving our kids to unhealthy habits?" The short answer is, "Yes!" The report card affirms that getting students moving to and from school is something we need to do better (Active Healthy Kids Canada, 2013). And it makes a big difference! Here is some key information from the report card:

- If children walked for all trips of less than 1 km rather than be driven, they would take an average of 2,238 more steps a day! This equates to between 15 and 20 minutes of physical activity a day—a substantial contribution to the 60 minutes per day that is recommended.

- Students who use active transportation to and from school average 45 minutes a day more of moderate to vigorous physical activity than those who take a train, car, or bus.
- While 58% of parents say they walked to school, only 28% of their children do now.

Obviously, we need to make a change. What can schools do? The report card has several key recommendations:

- **Parents and Guardians.** Encourage children to use active transportation to get to school as well as to friends' houses, playgrounds, and so on. Take turns with other parents to supervise children as needed. If you must drive, park some distance from your destination and walk to it. It's good for you, too!
- **Schools.** Place bike racks in visible areas. When constructing new schools, consider the location of racks from the perspective of children's travel needs. Actively facilitate "walking school busses" (adult volunteers accompanying students on walks to and from school), support active transport events, implement road safety education, and work with community partners to ensure safety.
- **Policy makers.** Consider the built environment and how it can facilitate activity for children. Implement and enforce traffic-calming measures in school communities. Work with employers to encourage flexible hours to enable parents to take their kids to school via active means.

Other questions about active transport that a healthy school community planning team should ask include:

- Does the school encourage and accommodate walking, biking, and inline skating by designating car-free zones and providing secure areas on school property to lock up bicycles, skates, skateboards, scooters, helmets, and protective padding?
- Do signs and electronic message boards convey messages promoting active transportation?
- Do the school's communication methods (newsletters, website, social media) identify and promote safe routes to and from school?
- Does the school organize "walk-to-school" days, walking or skipping clubs, or walking school busses?
- Are opportunities provided for school personnel to serve as role models in terms of active transportation?

SUCCESS STORY

Mohawk Gardens Public School—Reimagining a School Environment

By Christa Costas-Bradstreet, CCB Consulting, Burlington

My introduction to Mohawk Gardens Public School in Burlington, Ontario, actually took place before my children were born and attended school there. To get to know the area near our home, my husband and I would run in the neighbourhood, often passing by what we thought was a recently closed school. The oddly shaped building—it resembles a space station—proclaimed its name on a dirty, old sign. Overgrown bushes blocked part of the sign, as well as the view of one of the school entrances. Paint on the soffits was chipping. Blacktop in the fenced-in kindergarten area was cracked and surrounded by dirt. Two small circles of dirt on the front lawn contained a few plants, large rocks, and one tree with a memorial plaque, all overgrown with weeds. The area behind the school had broken basketball nets, a blacktop area that was uneven and cracked, and an old rusted tether-ball pole (with no ball) sticking from the ground. Farther behind the building next to the dumpster were bent and rusted bike racks. We soon came to learn that the school was in fact operating; however, having no children at the time, we did not think much about it other than to wonder what the future of this school might be.

Several years later I entered this school to attend junior kindergarten orientation for my first daughter. The orientation took place in the library—a warm and welcoming room. It had the feel and appearance of a sunken living room with stairs leading down from the school's main hallways and it was surrounded by bookshelves and lively decorations. However, the library's coziness could not disguise the rest of the school's aged and tired interior, which most noticeably included make-shift partitions (consisting in part of stacked boxes) to give individual classrooms some privacy and soundproofing. Despite these and other signs of aging, such as worn carpets, floors, and lockers, the classrooms themselves were creatively decorated and welcoming.

Mohawk Gardens Public School is very different today from when my husband and I first ran by it in 1992. The blacktop at the back of the school and in the kindergarten area has been repaired. Today it features game markings including several hopscotch-themed games, three four-square games, foot hockey courts, and a race track in the kindergarten area for special tricycles. The area has new play toys, as well as a shed in which to store all the new physical activity and gardening equipment. The space also features a kinderGARDEN—areas of flower beds with perennials and decorative stones, two planters with seasonal plants, and bird houses hanging from trees. The space was created primarily through volunteer time and donations as well as a small grant from a local horticultural association.

At the back of the school, basketball nets have been replaced and recess bins with different types of physical activity equipment to suit children of all ages have been replenished. The creative playground was expanded with specifically selected fitness-enhancing components. The bike racks (still old) were moved to the side of the school in the main blacktop area. According to one parent, "We moved the bike racks to a more prominent space and saw a huge increase in bike riding to school because not only are the bikes visible and students aware of them, they are also safer because the racks are in the open."

With the intention of beautifying the school, an environmental sub-committee conducted a walk-about and identified several ways to make Mohawk Gardens more attractive. The soffits have been painted and two large flower pots with seasonal foliage welcome visitors entering the front doors. A new, clean sign welcomes visitors, while the overgrown bushes have been removed. In their place is a new garden featuring a memorial tree and stone commemorating a Grade 4 student who passed away in 2006. Everyone agrees with the sentiment that "the school has changed in its appearance from the outside. It's becoming more and more beautiful to look at as you drive by."

Inside the school, one significant physical change is the conversion of a spare multipurpose room with dirty, worn carpeting and tired, dark paint into a bright, vibrant space for the school's snack program. The principal used school board funds to replace the carpeting with new tiles, while the caretaker secured some free paint that enabled a volunteer to repaint the room. A "Food for Thought" grant enabled the snack committee to buy new equipment, counter tops, sink, dishwasher, tables and chairs, and other supplies. A fridge has been donated. Bulletin boards mounted on the walls display menus, volunteer notices, and other postings. The room is decorated and children can enjoy donated toys and books while their parents or guardians are volunteering at the program.

A feature wall inside the school now boasts a lovely mural of people running. A teacher created the mural in a paint-by-numbers style that students then completed. Lockers have been painted, boxes of old files that for years sat atop the classroom dividers and shelves have been discarded, and new flooring has been installed. Classrooms are beautifully decorated and welcoming, as are the main foyer and office. Bulletin boards in all areas of the school highlight student achievements.

Parents, guardians, teachers, students, administration and support staff almost unanimously agreed that the school is clean, tidy, and attractive and the positive impact has benefited the school community from academic, psychological, and social perspectives. One teacher remarked that "the cleanliness of the building, the amount of organization, respect for where things go and how things work, the upkeep of the building and those kinds of things I would say have increased immensely over the years.... As we made the building a better place, it has instilled respect for things from the parents and the children as well, so that pride builds." ■

SUCCESS STORY

Belgravia Elementary School's Naturalization Project

By Kim Sanderson

Transforming a school's grounds supports children's growth and development at each step in the process. In the case of Belgravia Elementary School in Edmonton, children, parents, teachers, and community residents were integrally involved in a transformation project through planning and design, development, and now ongoing use and maintenance. Although the Belgravia initiative was a highly ambitious undertaking, transformations need not always be so. Greening projects can take a range of forms, from creating simple butterfly gardens and small garden plots, to planting trees and creating bird habitats.

This is how the Belgravia project came into being. One key at the beginning was recognizing the strategic importance of creating something that would have potential benefit for everyone.

- **Project organization.** The Belgravia project used a multi-layered approach, allowing everyone to participate at their comfort level. Care was taken to find ways to engage children meaningfully. Parents and guardians were asked to help provide overall project direction while the bulk of the work was carried out by a school greening committee made up of students, a teacher, and a parent. The general school community was called upon to perform various tasks throughout the process. Spreading out the authority and tasks allowed for greater involvement on the part of many participants, thus avoiding overtaxing any one individual or group.
- **Design and development.** The greening committee prepared, distributed, and collated a survey. Student members learned that, if they were to collect useful information, it was important to precede the survey with an educational video on greening possibilities. Survey results helped the committee identify priority projects, including a pond, birdhouses, quiet social spaces, a garden, and a giant sunflower bed. Having established these priorities or "program statement," the greening committee worked through a fun design session with a landscape architect who volunteered his services to create a detailed plan. The children were amazed that their input could actually become a plan that might result in sod being turned! The art teacher worked with Grade 3 students for more than a month to build a three-dimensional model of the finished project. They displayed the model in a school hallway along with

a suggestion box to invite feedback. Teams of students, parents, guardians, teachers, and community experts worked out the logistics for the pond, dock, and bridge. Others researched and sourced plant materials for the mountain and boreal forest regions of the site. After securing funding and approvals and preparing the base site, the general school population planted trees and shrubs, filled the pond, built the bird and bathhouses, and planted the giant sunflower bed.

- **Use and maintenance.** Students, teachers and, community members enthusiastically welcomed visitors to the opening of the site. Teachers held reading classes in the garden. Grade 5 students headed out to the country to gather animals and plants to stock the pond. Children played and roamed the garden during recess, after school, and on weekends. In the fall, wheat was harvested, threshed, and ground into flour to make bread. Pictures of giant sunflowers adorned the school walls and students took daily recordings of environmental changes to begin establishing a natural history of the site. The community even held a Play Day on the site to promote nature-based play and learning. What was once a flat, nondescript grassy space has been transformed into a special and beautiful place for people, plants, and animals.

The school put agreements in place to clearly outline roles and responsibilities for the site's continuing maintenance. During the summer, families look after the site for a week at a time. A steering group organizes cleaning days each spring and fall. Over the years, community individuals have adopted various parts of the site, working behind the scenes to make sure areas do not become overgrown. The project has evolved to meet the changing needs of teachers, students, parents, and the community. Each year there are more resources and workshop supports available for improving connections between the site and curriculum outcomes. Children who have been involved in the project from the beginning are proud of their legacy to the school and community. They never tire of the natural wonders that each season brings—or of simply being able to contemplate life on the dock before the school day begins. ■

The following table summarizes the many benefits inherent in projects dedicated to the naturalization of school grounds.

The Benefits of the Naturalization of School Grounds

For Students	For Teachers	For the School Community
• build environmental awareness • build a stronger sense of community • increase positive social interaction • speed recovery from mental fatigue • reduce stress • provide meaningful areas for playful learning • practise civility toward others • channel aggressive behaviours • situate the child within a caring community • reduce incidence of hostile behaviour • provide gender-neutral play spaces • instill greater school pride • provide opportunities to study plants, animals, and insects • add aesthetic value to the school grounds • foster understanding of diversity—respect for cultural differences and other creatures' needs • create a sense of place—introduce a sense of time and location • intensify investment in the school as a community, a family, a place where we live and learn together	• any topic or subject can come to life when a teacher plans lessons designed to enhance the hidden curriculum of school grounds • moving outdoors involves shifting from traditional teaching methods to more experiential methods • school ground transformation can be integrated into all aspects of curriculum • increased morale and enthusiasm for teaching • increased engagement and enthusiasm for learning • reduced discipline and classroom management problems	• greater opportunities for enriched connections with the community • greater opportunities for teachers to work together • greater opportunities for students across grades to work together • greater opportunities for schools engaged in similar projects to become partners • reduced disciplinary referrals, absenteeism, and dropout rates • reduced antisocial behaviour on school grounds • increased pride in school • a stronger sense of community • a chance to experience a community working together to make things better, help each other, and improve the conditions that optimize learning and caring.

Source: Adapted from Raffan, 2000.

Healthy Eating in Schools: Guidelines for Good Nutrition

Many jurisdictions now realize that we need to pay more attention to the types and quality of food we provide to children in schools, childcare facilities, and recreation/community facilities. This attention includes food rewards (candy for good behaviour), vending machines, fundraisers, and more—all with the goal of creating environments that support healthy food choices. For example, the Alberta Nutrition Guidelines for Children and Youth were developed in response to the declining quality of children's diets. Along with a variety of other continually evolving resources and supports, the guidelines and an accompanying school nutrition handbook provide concrete steps and supports for schools to address healthy eating. One of the most recognizable supports is a "traffic light" system by means of which foods are grouped into three categories:

- GREEN (GO!)—CHOOSE MOST OFTEN. These foods should be consumed daily in the amounts and portions recommended by Canada's Food Guide. Examples include fresh and frozen fruits and vegetables, lean meats, whole grains, and plain yogurt.
- YELLOW (YIELD!)—CHOOSE SOMETIMES. No more than three servings of these foods are recommended per week. Although they do provide some nutrients, these foods are higher in added sugar, salt, and unhealthy fats. Examples include canned fruits and vegetables with added sugar or salt, luncheon meat, enriched white breads, and flavoured fortified soy beverage.
- RED (STOP)—CHOOSE LEAST OFTEN. Limited to small portions and offered no more than once a week. Foods in this category are low in nutrients and high in calories, sugar, salt, and unhealthy fats. Examples include chips, sugared cereal, bakery items, and soda pop.

Canada's Food Guide and *Canada's Food Guide—First Nations, Inuit and Métis* are excellent examples of national guidelines that are readily accessible (both print and online) to schools, parents and guardians, and students.

Healthy Eating Spaces and Programs

Along with guidelines for *what* to serve and eat, we also need to consider *where* and *how* to support healthy eating in our schools.

Where?

- Are the school's layout, design, and kitchen or lunchroom facilities conducive to healthy food programs (such as breakfast, rainbow lunches, healthy snacks), food preparation, cooking, and communal meals?
- Does the school have an outdoor area where a patio, picnic tables, and barbecues could be set up?
- Do students have access to the following while eating: adequate number of tables and chairs, tables and chairs of appropriate height, drinking fountains in working order, a clean and inviting space, adequate supervision, servings of food grown at home or at school?
- Does the school offer healthy canteen/store and vending machine choices?

How?

- Does the school have an emergency food cupboard for students who forget to bring their lunch or do not have food from home for healthy lunches? Does the school provide support to students and their families who are experiencing issues related to food insecurity?
- What are the school's policies and procedures for dealing with disordered eating patterns?
- How does the school promote healthy food and beverage choices?
- Does the school encourage students to appreciate foods and meal customs of diverse cultures?
- Does the school provide opportunities for students to learn about healthy food preparation?
- Are healthy meal/snack preparation and healthy eating habits integrated into special events, festivities, celebrations, health fairs, talks by guest speakers, or family activity nights?
- Are physical activity initiatives and healthy eating programs combined and made part of your school's action plan? Do students understand the vital connection between physical activity and healthy eating?

Case Study

By Doug Gleddie

You have been offered a position (teacher, administrator, health worker—your choice) at an inner-city school starting in September. Well done! Or so you thought... When you move in to your new school in mid-August, you notice a few things:

- The school grounds consist mostly of broken concrete surfaces with a bit of greenery growing out of the cracks.
- The play structures should probably be condemned.
- When you walk through the main door, the first thing to catch your eye is a bank of vending machines—four of them in a row, with not a healthy choice to be found. There is no availability of healthy food on campus—at all.
- The gym is small and not well-ventilated and it seems to have been painted shortly after Confederation.
- The hallways have broken baseboards and loose tiles. There is water damage visible on ceiling tiles in some classrooms and many of the windows are screwed shut.

Fortunately, you just finished reading Chapter 4 of this book as part of your summer professional development activities. You decide to get to work to improve the physical environment of your new school using all the strategies and tools you have learned thus far.

1. Make a list of steps that you will take in your first year. What will your priorities be, and why? How will you decide what goals are achievable? How will you define and achieve success?
2. Knowing that it takes a community to build a healthy school, how will you involve all stakeholders in your vision for transformation? How will you convince the naysayers and the blockers? Who are the key partners in your community and how will you get them on board?
3. Change can be expensive. How will you raise funds for your school's healthy physical environment rejuvenation project? (Be specific, contextual, and detailed in your planning.)
4. Create a five-year plan of key steps that need to happen after the first year. Do not get bogged down in details. Think big and use information from this chapter to help develop a plan for all aspects of your healthy school transformation plan.

It's Your Turn

1 Initiate a school-wide assessment of your school involving students, parents, guardians, and staff. (Consider using the Healthy School Planner described in Chapter 2.) Include space for physical activity, outdoor learning, social-emotional learning, activities conducive to mental health (such as yoga, tai chi, or regular recess), healthy eating, community engagement, contemplation, and more! Make a visual display of your results, post them at a parent-teacher night, and invite everyone to add notes suggesting how they could use and improve these spaces.

2 Create a small committee to summarize results of the assessment and share the report with the school community for feedback and ratification. Prioritize ideas in terms of short-, medium-, and long-term goals and begin to work on a five-year implementation plan. Search for local, provincial, and federal grants and other funding sources (such as the parent council and school fundraisers) that might help you reach your goals.

✓ Action Checklist

Individual	Suggested Follow-up
Pre-service Teacher	❑ Talk with your peers and begin to accumulate a list of success stories that you experienced during your practicum. ❑ Share these stories with your mentor teacher and try to start a small project together in the time you have. ❑ Take time to meet with administration to solicit advice on funding sources and mechanisms for healthy school change.
Health and Physical Education Teacher	❑ Consider how the physical environment at the school can help achieve your HPE outcomes. ❑ Advocate for safe and engaging spaces where students can play, be active, and socialize. ❑ Connect with your community to share facilities and to improve activity space (e.g., outdoor rinks and playgrounds).
Administrator	❑ Consider a SWOT scan of your school's physical environment. What are its strengths? weaknesses? opportunities? threats? ❑ Create a multi-stakeholder committee to address your findings and assist in making a plan for improvement.
Parent/Guardian	❑ Consider what skills can be found in the parent community: hands-on trades, grant writing, advocacy, public speaking and media outreach, gardening, and so on. ❑ Develop a plan to improve the school's physical environment.
Health Promotion Coordinator	❑ Volunteer to coordinate the community aspect of the physical environment. ❑ Provide support for healthy eating with vending machine renewal or a healthy school store that sells produce from a greenhouse garden.

Chapter 4 Summary

Viewed as care for self and others, health should also be viewed as care for the environment. Health-promoting schools help students recognize the importance of caring for the school's physical setting and the surrounding natural environment, and the symbiotic relationship between the body and the environment. For example, walking or cycling to school is not only beneficial for physical health (such as cardiorespiratory fitness), but it also benefits the environment. Eating locally grown fruits and vegetables not only is a healthy food choice, it also helps reduce gas emissions from food trucks that travel thousands of miles. A recycling program at a school can help ensure that playgrounds are free from litter and debris while also reducing the amount of waste in landfills. Choices that are healthy for the environment often result in positive benefits for the body as well.

Showing care for the safety features, physical appearance, aesthetics, functionality, and accessibility of school environments not only enhances the physical health of the entire school community, but also elevates school spirit and reinforces community pride. Mobilizing stakeholders to improve school grounds and interiors provides opportunities for community building and creative problem solving.

Questions for Reflection

1 How can school staff and administrators strike a balance between welcoming visitors and encouraging community involvement in school activities and events while at the same protecting students from potentially dangerous situations or intruders?

2 What might constitute the most effective policies and strategies for promoting healthy eating both at school and at home?

3 Who are potential activists for school naturalization?

4 In your opinion, what are the three most significant benefits of school naturalization?

5 Schools that have undergone a naturalization process have more trees, shrubs, rocks/boulders, wildflower gardens, horticultural gardens, butterfly gardens, sand, logs, berms, water features, and food gardens. Some have a woodland habitat, grassland habitat, wetland habitat, greenhouses, nature trails, and composting stations. All are enhanced with birdfeeders, nesting structures for birds, art integrated with nature, gathering areas (reading zones, story circles, and platform/stage features for teaching outdoors). What would your schoolyard design look like if you included a water feature, gardens, and gathering areas? Create a plan on paper illustrating your ideal schoolyard naturalization.

6 If you wished to design a rock garden for your school that reflects the geological diversity of Canada, what kinds of community support could you enlist?

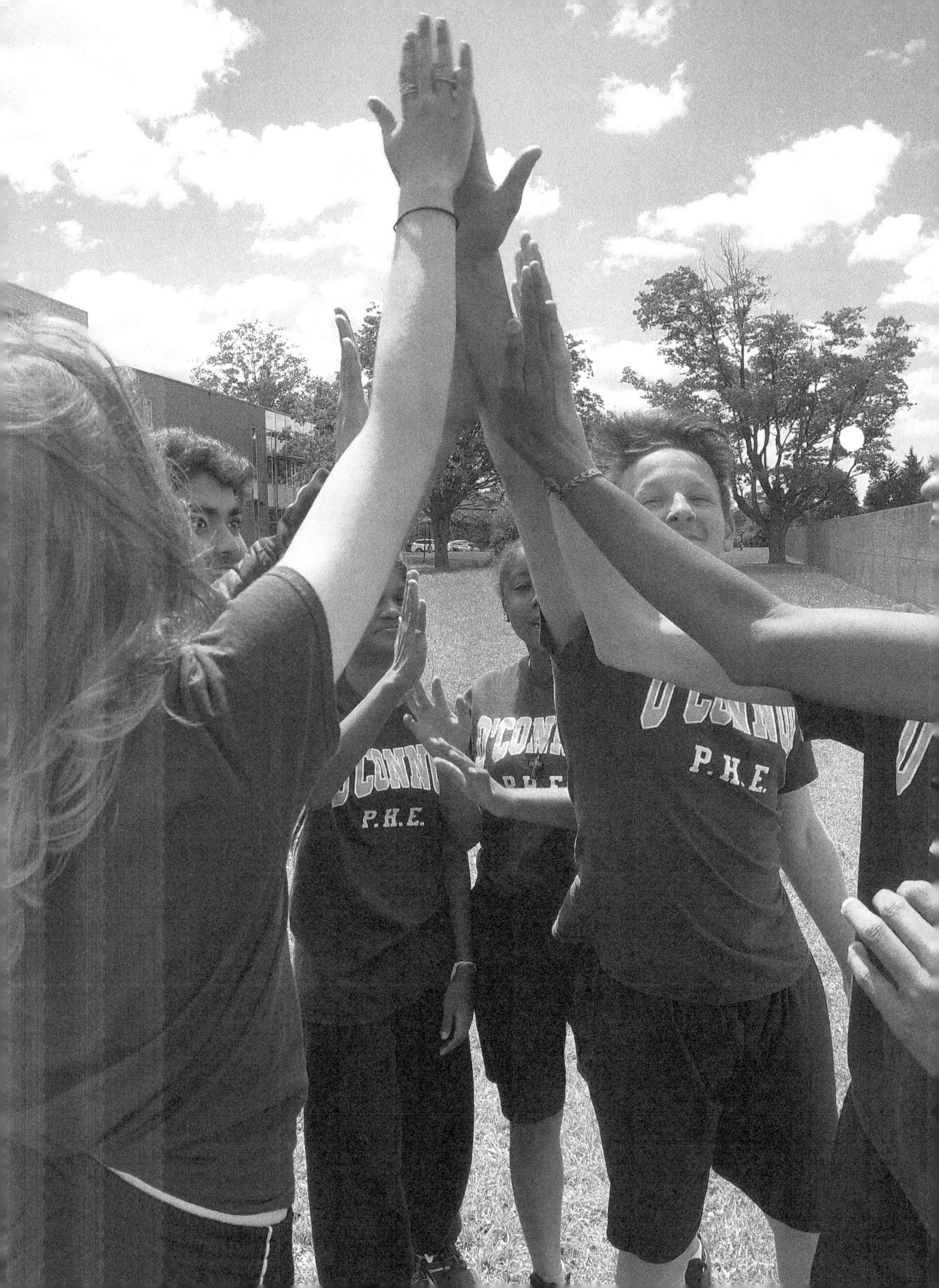
P.H.E.

5

The Social Environment of Health-Promoting Schools

Feeling empowered

Creating a school environment in which students feel healthy and nurtured contributes to the third important pillar of a health-promoting school. To be successful learners, students need to feel emotionally and physically safe, supported, encouraged, and empowered to make healthy decisions. This chapter highlights the importance of a school environment that supports the physical, psychological, and social development of students. Examples that showcase a positive school culture demonstrate the impact that a positive social and physical environment can have on the health and well-being of students.

A positive school culture refers to the overall social and physical atmosphere of a school as reflected in interpersonal relationships—how people greet each other in hallways, treat one another socially, participate in decision making, and so on. In other words, a healthy school culture is accepting and inclusive, and provides opportunities for everyone—students, parents, guardians, teachers, and other staff members—to learn and to grow. A school's culture is reflected not only in daily practices, rituals, and traditions. It is reflected as well on special occasions when members of the school community gather to commemorate annual events, celebrate student achievements in sports or the arts, or honour members of the community who are connected in a vital way to the school. A school's culture is evident in every corner of the building. For example, a cafeteria or lunch room can send clear messages about a school's support for healthy eating. Classrooms, hallways, gymnasiums, learning resource centres, administrative offices, and entrances to the school communicate a great deal about how the school is run, about the importance attached to student safety, and about school pride. If students could design school entranceways and corridors, what messages would they wish to convey to visitors and to each other about the accomplishments, talents, and values celebrated in their school?

Transforming a School's Culture

As you read the situations described here, consider the culture that each situation reflects and whether that culture supports and nurtures student and teacher learning and collaboration. What subtle messages are communicated by means of language, norms, and rituals? What implicit messages about control are communicated, and in what ways?

Situation 1
At one school students referred to the librarian as "Conan the Librarian" (named after a gladiator-type movie role). Students entering the library were greeted with reprimands for late returns. Concern with due dates overshadowed any encouragements the librarian might have given to students to explore the library's selections and to choose something fun and informative to read.

Situation 2
Students in a Grade 4 mathematics class were asked: "What are the important things to remember when completing this math assignment?" Students replied: "It's important to remember to use a pencil, not a pen.... Always put the date in the top right-hand corner.... Always start at the margin and keep the numbers in a straight line." It was startling to see how little students talked about any kind of authentic learning related to mathematics!

Situation 3
In a physical education class, students formed a line to take their turn high jumping. By the time all 32 students had had a second turn, the class was over. Why would the teacher organize the class in such a way? Do teachers in other subject areas expect an entire class to line up to use a single computer or a single book? What was the teacher more concerned about—effective instruction or exercising control over the students?

Invitational Education

One approach to creating a school culture that supports the development of a positive social environment is invitational education. "Invitational education is both a philosophy and set of activities intended to create a school climate that is welcoming; a place that intentionally stimulates people, helping them realize their individual and collective potential" (Friedland, 1999: p.14).

> ***Through the use of invitational education, students develop a strong connection to others. Actively engaging students in the learning process provides them with a sense of ownership and connectedness to real-life issues.*** —Key Assumptions of Invitational Education (adapted from Friedland, 1999).

In each situation described above, how could the teacher have demonstrated a more invitational approach?

For the librarian, getting to know students and their interests could help students identify books and other resources relevant to their daily lives—resources that the students might find useful or inspiring. For example, upon learning that a Grade 2 student had a new baby sister, the librarian could provide a selection of books that describe welcoming a new brother or sister into the family. Perhaps a student in Grade 5 has recently immigrated to Canada and is homesick. The student might appreciate gaining access to some books, magazines, or websites featuring images from their home country.

For the mathematics teacher, an important component of numeracy is assessment of math concepts. A typical "assessment of learning" question about the value of money might be: "If you have three dimes, five quarters, and five one-dollar coins, how much money do you have?" This type of question may help assess students' basic knowledge of the value of coins; however, it does not help students understand the value of money. An invitational approach to assessment might involve asking the question: "Think of three different combinations of coins that each totals $2.65. If you had $2.65 for lunch each day, what could you buy?" The teacher could also point out to students that humanitarian organizations such as Plan International and UNICEF have programs in developing countries that encourage monetary donations for specific projects. For example, a $17 donation to Plan International provides a family with baby chicks that will eventually lay eggs and provide a source of food and income for the family. If everyone in the class has $2.65, how many donations of baby chicks could the class make?

For the physical education teacher, setting up various fitness stations for a class could encourage optimal challenges for students while also maximizing time on task. The stations could be arranged to require minimal supervision and to offer various levels of challenges by letting students choose the level of difficulty of the task. For example, a student could choose from a list of three yoga poses that vary in levels of difficulty but that still help develop core strength.

Invitational teaching helps students make connections to their day-to-day lives and encourages the use of assessment as learning. The ways in which we assess students can have a lasting impact on their psychosocial health.

Although the intent of the examiner in the cartoon shown on the following page may be to assess each animal's ability to climb, the assessment chosen is not representative of each animal's climbing skills. For example, to survive, the penguin and the seal must be able to navigate terrains of snow and ice to avoid potential predators. Trees cannot even grow in many of the habitats in which these animals live!

While the scenario in this cartoon is intentionally exaggerated for the sake of humour, off-target and ineffectual assessments can have long-lasting negative consequences on the psychosocial health of students. Take fitness testing, for example. A physical education teacher may decide to use a beep test to assess students' cardiovascular fitness. In a beep test, students run between two lines 20 metres apart, attempting to cover the distance before a pre-recorded beep sounds. A student who fails to reach the opposite line before the beep sounds is eliminated. As the test progresses,

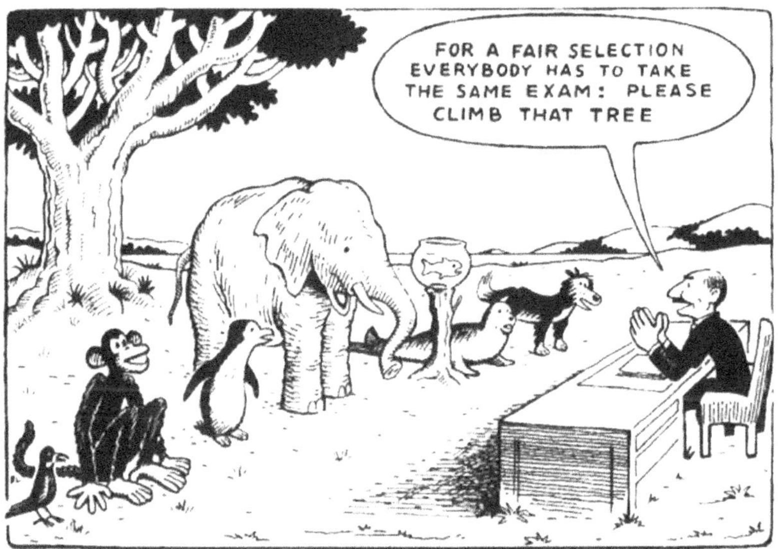

the time interval between beeps is shortened, thus gradually eliminating students from the test. A student's cardiorespiratory fitness is measured by comparing their elimination time to a normative set of data collected about students of the same age and gender. If a student who is less fit is eliminated at the beginning of this test in front of peers, that student's psychosocial experience cannot be described as a positive one!

What if a teacher were to use an invitational approach to teaching and assessing cardiorespiratory health instead? The teacher could engage students in a classroom discussion about the importance of cardiorespiratory health, inviting them to identify personal benefits such as increased energy, reduced bouts of sickness, and better concentration in school. If they wish, they might also discuss personal experiences involving cardiorespiratory health, such as having a relative who suffers from heart disease or a respiratory condition. The teacher could guide students in researching some of the social and economic costs of cardiorespiratory disease and discuss ways to promote heart health through appropriate nutrition and regular physical activity. In doing so, the teacher provides a context for why everyone's cardiorespiratory health is important. Students may begin to wonder about the status of their own cardiorespiratory health. That opens up a conversation about ways in which students might assess their own heart health. Students could discuss the pros and cons of each method, how they might use the information obtained from each assessment, or which assessment they might prefer to use. The result of this invitational approach to learning about cardiorespiratory health is a much broader understanding of the importance of heart health in ways that are comparatively more personalized, more respectful, and more choice-based. Additionally, they are more conducive to students' psychosocial health because they do not expose students to scrutiny and embarrassment if they do not "ace" only one assessment of many—the beep test—that might not be suitable for everyone.

An Ethic of Care as a Moral Compass

When we teach any subject, we link it to areas of care. For example, in a discussion of social and economic barriers to healthy living, questions such as the following often arise:

- How does discrimination interfere with opportunities to lead a healthy life?
- How does respect for others affect feelings of self-worth and efforts to be healthy?
- What does it mean to live in an inclusive community that encourages healthy living for everyone?

For our schools, an ethic of care is a moral compass, helping us to think strategically about what and how we do things. The organizational and management structures that we encourage through policy making serve to build relationships that intensify and expand the knowledge and skills needed to a) develop health-promoting programs, b) create emotionally and physically safe environments, and c) build mutually beneficial relationships with support services and partners. By facilitating policies and processes that encourage problem solving, critical thinking, planning, and analysis of situations in relation to quality of life, students begin to develop a richer sense of the importance of care for others as well as care for the environment.

Education is about providing experiences that contribute to the overall development of young people as learners, citizens, and agents for change. An emphasis on health promotion humanizes education. Deeply rooted in the practice of health is an ethic of care. A moral purpose guides who students aspire to be, what they do, and how they relate to others. Indeed, the goal of health is to achieve self-actualization and happiness through ethical goals and deeds. Service to self is actually unselfish because it is our duty to society to build our potential to contribute as citizens, family members, and participants in communities. Service to others is our gift to the soul.

An ethic of care has obvious parallels to "service learning," an educational approach that combines classroom instruction with meaningful community service. A goal-setting and action process that affects others positively, service learning encourages critical thinking, personal reflection, a strong sense of community, civic engagement, and personal responsibility.

Service learning creates opportunities for students to accomplish the following:

- strengthen academic knowledge and skills by applying them to real-life issues
- build positive relationships
- discover new interests and abilities
- set and achieve goals
- work together
- become leaders
- learn the value of helping and caring for others
- create a sense of belonging
- develop a positive sense of self

Service learning goes beyond service projects to offer students opportunities to better understand the purpose and value of their efforts through the practical experience of serving in the community. It contributes to welcoming, caring, respectful, and safe learning environments by providing opportunities for students and staff to work together on common causes. Types of hands-on learning that constitute service learning include volunteerism, community service, internships, and field education.

Psychosocial Development and Quality of Life

Schools can become a place where students' psychosocial development is enhanced when teaching and learning prioritize health promotion. Socially cohesive and democratic school cultures instill in students a sense of school membership through which they experience feelings of communal acceptance, belonging, and attachment to school life. Environmental conditions shape individual students' feelings and attitudes that, in turn, can directly affect each student's academic performance, mental health, and behaviour (McCall, 2004).

> According to Kohn (1996), seeing the school as a community means that:
> ***". . . it is a place in which students feel cared about and are encouraged to care about each other. They experience a sense of being valued and respected; the children matter to one another and to the teacher. They have come to think in the plural; they feel connected to each other; they are part of an 'us' and, as a result of all this, they feel safe in their classes, not only physically but emotionally."*** (pp.101–102).

WHO's quality-of-life model encourages organizations to examine the factors that contribute to the goodness and meaning of life and, ultimately, to people's health. This model guides program development and implementation, as well as research. It portrays life experiences and school activities in terms of three domains: being, belonging, and becoming (Renwick & Brown, 1996). Each domain has three categories.

- Being relates to who one is and this category is divided into the physical, the psychological, and the spiritual. Physical being includes physical health, personal hygiene, nutrition, exercise, grooming, clothing, and general physical appearance. Psychological being focuses on psychological health and adjustment, cognitions, feelings, self-esteem, self-concept, and self-control. Spiritual being embraces personal values, standards of conduct, and spiritual beliefs.
- Belonging relates to connections with our environments. This domain is divided into physical, social, and community belonging. Physical belonging concerns places such as the home, workplace, school, neighbourhood, and community. Social belonging involves relationships with intimate others (family, friends, and perhaps co-workers), people in our neighbourhoods, and community life.

Community belonging involves having an adequate income and access to health and social services, employment, educational programs, recreational programs, and community events and activities.

- Becoming relates to achieving personal goals, dreams, and aspirations. This category is divided into practical, leisure, and growth areas. Practical becoming concerns domestic activities, paid work, school or volunteer activities, and taking care of health or social needs. Leisure becoming concerns activities that promote relaxation and stress reduction. Growth becoming focuses on activities that promote the maintenance or improvement of knowledge and skills, as well as adaptation to change.

Providing children with opportunities at school to develop those characteristics associated with quality of life will help children who struggle at home. Many children in Canada live in unfavourable or deprived conditions. According to a UNICEF report (Adamson, 2016), of the world's 29 wealthiest countries, Canada ranked only 17th in terms of child well-being. On measures of health inequality and life satisfaction for children, Canada's position dropped to 24th of 35 countries surveyed. Schools can play a critical role in helping to improve these scores and reduce inequities. In a health-promoting school, students are encouraged to dream, to express ideas and hopes, to strive for success, and to learn that aspirations matter. A caring environment can make an enormous difference in a child's life.

Educators who value, respect, and empower students can help them to become healthy, effective risk-takers who readily engage in the learning process. To achieve something close to this optimal state of affairs, teachers must strive to adopt a positive approach in everything they do. Here are some practical suggestions for how teachers can foster positive psychosocial behaviours and outcomes in their schools.

Create a Sense of Being

- Work frequently with students to help them acquire decision-making skills. Encourage them to examine alternatives, decide on a course of action, act upon their decision, recognize consequences, and evaluate whether the decision is one they would choose again.
- Plan with students various tools to record and measure their own progress, such as daily verbal or written feedback, weekly scores, time records, self-assessment checklists, journals describing growth or progress, a wall chart in the classroom to record books they have read, a tally sheet of positive interactions with others, and so on.
- Review with children the impact they have on others or the changes that occur because of their suggestions, initiatives, or efforts. Help them see that determination to set and achieve prosocial goals can bring about positive change.
- Adopt a problem-solving approach to issues to help students learn to manage their own responses by using a consistent approach to define an issue, examine the factors that caused the issue, explore various options to resolve the issue, and select and apply a course of action.

- Ask parents and guardians to provide positive and constructive feedback to their child with respect to changes they see at home or observations about their child's growth and development.
- Provide opportunities for children to display their accomplishments through various media—a talent show, a dramatic reading or play, a blog, a puppet show, a video or electronic slide show, a composition, a drawing, an evaluative summary, a bulletin board, a website posting, and so on.
- Post coloured signs in the classroom to indicate the standards of behaviour expected during any given activity. For example, a blue sign might indicate that children can talk quietly with their neighbours or move around as they work. Yellow might represent a time frame during which movement is limited. Red might indicate that students are not to talk or move around the room for a while in order to provide some quiet reading or reflection time.
- Counsel students who seem intent on attracting attention. Confer with each student to develop a list of acceptable ways to get attention when they need it. Such a list might include regular opportunities for oral sharing in class, a one-on-one session with a teacher aide or guidance counsellor, and pairing work with a partner.
- Set aside time at the end of each day or each week for students to evaluate their class's behaviour, note growth, express appreciation for others' ideas and contributions, and set goals for the future.
- Teach children about how they either hurt or help others by the comments they make. Encourage them to develop their skills in communicating wisely and assertively rather than aggressively, passively, or heedlessly.
- Provide opportunities for children to serve in leadership capacities. Children need to learn to lead, take responsibility for those they lead, and be accountable for the responsibilities delegated to them.
- Deal with violations or problems on a one-on-one basis whenever possible to avoid embarrassing students in front of their peers. Avoid sarcasm or teasing when dealing with infractions. Always end on an optimistic note or with a word of encouragement.
- Provide small cards to children who have difficulty remembering not to talk, to stay in their seats, or to observe other classroom rules. List on each card the rules on which the student needs to focus.
- Create a large bulletin board or display area that can be divided into sections to provide each student with space to post worksheets, creative writing, photos, or artwork. Have children take all their material home at the end of the week or month. Then, start over.
- Encourage diversity in thinking processes. Explain that students must arrive at their own decisions on many questions rather than be led by the opinions of others. Have them practise with their peers the concept of accepting and not being judgmental about the viewpoints of others. Plan debates on issues in which different points of view can be justified by specific facts and logical arguments rather than vague opinions or biases.

- Schedule time each week to work individually with each student. Use the time to offer encouragement, recognize growth, or discuss worries or fears the child might express.
- Give children opportunities to meet privately with you to explain any personal problems they are facing in their daily lives and how they are learning to cope with them.
- Set up a personal mailbox and invite students to address notes to the teacher; give feedback on how their day went; express frustration, anxiety, or fear; or ask a question to clarify something about which they feel uncomfortable or uncertain.
- Use both classical music and popular songs as vehicles for helping children get in touch with their moods and feelings. Follow up a listening session with a discussion about experiences such as how students felt when they started attending a new school, when they received a birthday card in the mail, when a pet died, when they lost a friend, when someone teased them, or when other significant personal events occurred. Use the discussion as a starting point for writing activities.
- Use activity centres, discovery days, or exploratoriums (special afternoons) to expand students' horizons by offering them a chance to investigate new ideas or skills, or learn about a topic that intrigues them.
- Invite parents, guardians, or other members of the community to visit your class to share their interests, hobbies, or collections. Visits such as these serve to encourage children to develop their own special interests. Topics might include painting, drawing, colouring, scrapbooking, photography, carving, coin or stamp collecting, building model trains or airplanes, computer applications, cooking, tool use, sewing, and ceramic work.
- Use puppets in role-playing to help young children act out real-life situations. Have students use the puppets to depict incidents that occurred in the playground and express how they felt in those situations.
- Have each child help you plan a conference with their parent or guardian. Use part of the conference to allow the student to demonstrate new skills and areas of growth about which the child is proud.

Create a Sense of Belonging

- Provide opportunities for students to work together in small groups or as a class. Assign tasks that involve working with a partner by pairing students who have difficulty with those who can help them so that everyone can feel successful.
- Make special efforts to welcome new students. Assign a buddy to accompany each new student to school during their first week or two. Create a special bulletin board for new students (if they wish) to introduce themselves by listing or illustrating their interests and background experiences.
- Build class pride through cooperative team efforts—start a garden, decorate the classroom or school foyer, throw a surprise party for the school custodian or educational assistant, adopt a pet, clean up the schoolyard, challenge another class in a fundraising competition, make a class banner or class buttons, raise money for a field trip, plan an overnight camping trip, and so on.

- Find ways to provide positive recognition for students who isolate themselves from others without forcing others to be with them. For example, have these students assign use of balls or other equipment at recess, dispense privileges, or serve as tutors in the skills in which they excel or in which they have been coached.
- Create cards or buttons that state, "I appreciate what you did today." Use them and encourage students to use them as well to recognize others for their contributions or support.
- Appoint a resource person for each child who is struggling so that they have someone to whom they can go for help or tutoring. Depending on the situation, this person could be a peer mentor, a parent/guardian volunteer, or a staff member. This system may relieve the teacher and encourage service to others. Monitor this system to see that no individual is over-burdened or overly dependent.
- Assign responsibilities to different members of the class to encourage a feeling of belonging. Responsibilities might include taking roll call, recording homework, looking after pets, watering plants, setting up bulletin board displays, greeting visitors, and cleaning up.
- Label positive social behaviour in specific terms. Rather than admonishing children to "be good," compliment specific acts: "Picking up Ramos's book was a kind thing to do," or "Sharing your laptop was generous and thoughtful."
- Assign children to small play or study teams. Have students choose a name or a symbol for their group to give the group an identity. Encourage them to help each other in activities and projects such as research, web explorations, art projects, murals, math games, thinking activities, spelling, or reading to one another.
- Draw names for secret pals. Encourage each child to help their pal feel good about themselves at least once every day through sharing something to eat (after checking with the teacher to ensure there is no risk of food allergies or sensitivities), offering help with homework, sharing funny jokes or stories, including the secret pal in a game, or passing on a compliment.
- Plan a time for students to teach others a new skill or pass on information they have learned that would be of general interest, such as how to play a new game or sport, how to play an instrument, how to build something, or how to cook.
- Introduce students to non-competitive sports in which everyone can feel themselves to be a part of the team. Use movement exploration activities frequently to build skills and de-emphasize competition.
- Have a class of older students adopt a primary grade class, serving occasionally as tutors or aides to help with story-writing or reading. Select students from time to time to read their stories to the primary class. Have the younger students dictate stories to their assigned older partners.

SUCCESS STORY

Treeline Public School

By Carol Scaini

Building a healthy school takes more than just eating healthy foods and being active. It requires developing a deeper understanding of what it means to be healthy. It means creating a sense of belonging, of participating at and contributing to our school, our neighbourhood, our community, and our world—to help create a better place for all of us to live.

Treeline Public School in Brampton, Ontario, adopted the comprehensive school health (CSH) model to bring into focus new ways of thinking about curriculum, to improve learning, and, ultimately, to improve the overall health of our students. By means of a range of initiatives, we are creating opportunities for students, parents and guardians, school staff, and community partners to work together to pursue sustainable healthy living.

Our school strives to create and sustain a learning environment that promotes mental, physical, spiritual, and emotional health in our classrooms and that will extend to our school community and beyond. Our aim is to teach, nurture, and inspire young minds with ideas, understanding, and leadership opportunities. We encourage students to become self-directed learners who are challenged and motivated to reach beyond their limits.

Our CSH team has developed projects and outreach programs at the individual, community, and global levels. We promote a health-education program to help students acquire the knowledge, attitudes, and skills needed to live a healthy lifestyle (e.g., by understanding and applying *Canada's Food Guide* in their daily lives and by learning about the effects of appropriate nutritional choices).

We also provide students with a variety of open-ended experiences that foster independence, resourcefulness, competence, and self-confidence. Health lessons, for example, foster children's natural enthusiasm for problem solving, allowing them to take risks, make mistakes, persevere, explore all possibilities and alternative strategies, and devise creative solutions to unique situations.

The programs in our school go beyond the classroom. On an environmental level, for example, our staff and students have teamed up with our parent council and a local sports equipment company to purchase outdoor equipment (including fun hoops and basketball hoops) and to paint lines on an asphalt surface for playing recreational games such as hopscotch and four-square. We have partnered with a local home renovation company to revitalize our school's natural environment by planting trees, building planters at the school entrance, and inviting parents and guardians to donate flower bulbs. In addition, we installed an outdoor classroom for our staff and students to take their learning outside.

Our recycling team encouraged classes to reduce the amount of garbage we produce and to help keep our community clean and litter-free. One of our classrooms achieved the goal of reducing waste to a volume of 500 mL or less each day. Our Green Team empowered our students to reduce our carbon footprint with a walk to school program. Each Friday, they celebrated those students who walk to school with a "Footloose Friday" ballot to win some environmentally friendly prizes each month. These prizes include such items as reusable water bottles and lunch containers, sporting equipment, and Treeline t-shirts. In partnership with Peel Health, we have implemented the "5-2-1-0" initiative to promote healthy living for all staff, students and their families. This initiative included eating 5 servings of fruit and vegetables; participating in 2 hours or less of screen time; being active for 1 hour of exercise and consuming 0 sugar-sweetened beverages each day.

These and other initiatives demonstrate our firm commitment to live according to the four pillars of the CSH model.

Our school community is proud of our accomplishments and we continue to focus on linking health education to life beyond the school. By thinking outside the box, we have developed outreach programs that foster a rich sense of what it means to be part of a community that values all people. At Treeline Public School, each grade is responsible for focusing on a health component in our community. Although each grade has a specific focus, the project is collaborative because no one group "owns" any initiative.

Our primary students (K–3) are establishing the foundation of character education and healthy living for themselves. As part of their program, they participate in some of the healthy-living programs initiated by students in other grades.

Grade 4 students partnered with our local Punjabi Cultural Community Services and the Salvation Army to provide food baskets for families in need. Through the leadership of these students and their teachers, the entire school community managed to fill more than 40 baskets.

Grade 5 students worked with senior citizens in our local seniors' centre. They planned opportunities for social interaction—playing cards and bingo, singing, and enjoying arts and crafts with seniors. In return, many seniors shared their talents with our students. As a long-lasting benefit, some students continue to exchange letters with the seniors they met.

Grade 6 students took part in Variety Village's Outreach ability awareness program. This hands-on program promotes diversity, inclusion, integration, and active living through adapted sport and recreation. Students participated in modified hockey and wheelchair basketball activities and spoke with individuals about the implications of living with their disability.

Grade 7 students held a food drive at school and then visited the Toronto Daily Bread Food Bank to donate the food they collected and to volunteer for the day. This experience allowed them to examine the need for ongoing food donations and the importance of helping others. During a competition between classes to bring in the most canned goods, one student acknowledged that it did not matter who won. Everyone wins when we do our part.

Finally, Grade 8 students are working toward understanding global health issues. As part of the critical literacy component of our Language Arts program, students are focusing on poverty and its implications. Providing students with an opportunity to interpret and debate issues, such as poverty and child labour, helps them develop a deeper understanding of these societal issues. Students joined Oprah Winfrey's Ambassadors/Free the Children program, with the goals of raising awareness of issues facing communities in South Asia and raising money to help improve living conditions in that part of the world. As most of Treeline's families have roots in South Asia, this afforded students an opportunity to make connections on an international level and to help make a major difference in people's lives.

With the increased focus on mental health, our Grade 8 students have also been learning about various strategies and technique to use during stressful times to help them cope. With this knowledge, our Grade 8s have been paired up, and then partnered with, one of our Kindergarten to Grade 7 classes. Once a week, during our Daily Physical Activity time, the Grade 8s take on a leadership role and present a "Mindful Minute" to their particular class. The "Mindful Minute" sessions include breathing and meditation techniques students may use during stressful situations.

As a staff, we introduced a "Caught Being Kind" ticket to capture our students who demonstrate one of Peel's character attributes: honest, respectful, caring, responsible, inclusive, and cooperative behaviour. The top portion of the ticket goes home so the child's family can celebrate their child's excellence, while the bottom portion of the ticket is posted on our Caught Being Kind thermometer in the hallway. It is wonderful to see the hundreds of wonderful deeds our students do to enrich the lives of others throughout the year. Our staff has a similar way to acknowledge each other. We have a corkboard in our administrative hallway where we post notes to thank our colleagues for their kindness and support for each other. By celebrating all of these little things, together we celebrate the excellence that is Treeline Public School.

Adopting the CHS framework at Treeline Public School has allowed us to engage students in relevant and meaningful hands-on, interactive experiences. This has inspired them to take ownership of their own health and well-being. Providing them with the necessary tools, skills, and confidence to make healthy life choices has empowered them to think and act creatively and to transfer "knowing" health-related skills to "doing" healthy actions. ■

Create a Sense of Becoming

- Make a list of things children might want to learn. Have them select areas that would interest them, skills they would like to acquire, topics they would like to explore, and experiences they would like to try. Encourage them to set a goal or objective based upon their interests and plan how they might achieve it.
- Have children compile a list of skills they have already acquired, such as proficiency in grammar, math, and reading, as well as social and physical skills. Then have them list additional skills that they need to work on next and use this list as a basis for setting goals.
- Have students define their dreams. What kind of person would they like to become? What skills would they like to have as an adult? How would they like to be seen by others? For which acts would they like to be recognized? Help them select some short-term and long-term goals on which they might work to help them achieve their dreams.
- Provide opportunities for children to experience different forms of music, art, drama, poetry, and other means of expression. Expose them to the works of great artists and musicians. Share with them some of the problems and challenges that artists have had to overcome to reach their goals. Encourage children to broaden their ability to express their feelings and ideas through different media and art forms.
- Discuss lifestyles, life goals, and a wide variety of occupations. Inform students about the levels of training and education needed for each occupation, as well as the rewards and benefits associated with each one. Emphasize that the accumulation of wealth is not an end in itself but rather a means to actualize human potential. Help students research and discuss the types of occupations that appeal to them.
- Express confidence in each student's ability to succeed. Encourage students to strive to meet challenges, and convey faith in their ability to do so. Children need to feel the constant support of someone who believes in them.
- Create an atmosphere that encourages children to strive for new levels of proficiency. Challenge them to try to attain a higher level in reading or to work on more complex math problems without feeling defeated if they do not succeed. Help them learn how to benefit from their mistakes and to view learning as a valuable experience involving trial and error.
- Provide opportunities for children to develop a personal profile of skills using diagnostic testing or a skills inventory to determine their current level of achievement. The profile can be used as a basis for appropriate individualized learning targets.
- When giving assignments to students, explain their purpose. Help children see the relevance of the work they are doing, the usefulness of the skills they are expected to develop, the validity of the knowledge they are expected to acquire, and the significance of the connections they can make between their learning and the world beyond the school. How might this work relate to making a difference in people's lives?

Psychosocial Health and Mental Well-Being

The stakes associated with ensuring positive psychosocial health in our schools and communities have never been greater. Although significant progress has occurred in reducing the stigma associated with mental illness, the availability of support mechanisms to foster positive mental health still lags behind demand. Highlights of the 2015 Ontario Student Drug Use and Health Survey (Boak et al., 2015) of students in Grades 7 to 12 reveal that:

- The percentage of students who rated their mental health as fair to poor increased from 11% in 2007 to 17% in 2015.
- One in eight students had seriously considered suicide while 3% of those surveyed reported a suicide attempt during the previous year.
- Significantly more students in 2015 than in 2013 reported symptoms such as anxiety or depression related to a moderate to serious level of psychological distress.
- 28% of students reported that they wanted to talk to someone about a mental health problem but did not know whom to approach.
- Almost twice as many students in 2015 reported visiting a mental health professional compared to students in 1999.

Supporting Minds is a reference document that the Ontario Ministry of Education published in 2012 to help educators support students who are struggling with mental health issues and to promote positive mental health. This resource recognizes that "Mental health exists on a continuum and can be enhanced through positive relationships with supportive friends, congenial social opportunities, involvement in meaningful activities, and the effective management of stress and conflict" (p.16). Supporting Minds offers an extensive overview of strategies to support vulnerable students and to foster an inclusive and safe environment that promotes positive mental health. A positive school climate that offers these supports will have "programs and activities that focus on the building of healthy relationships, a safe, inclusive, and accepting learning environment, character development, and positive peer relations" (Ontario Ministry of Education, 2012, p.2).

Open lines of communication within a school that allow students to feel comfortable discussing mental health issues not only help break down stigma, but also help reassure those students with a mental health problem that they are not alone.

Positive Social, Emotional, and Mental Health

Schools are vitally important in promoting positive mental health: a growing number of educators, parents, and community members recognize the significant role that mental health plays in learning—and in life! A JCSH report by Morrison and Peterson in 2013 includes several key assumptions that frame values common to education and health that can foster positive mental health in children and youth. These include:

- Child and youth engagement and empowerment are critical considerations for facilitating positive development or change (p.8).

- Children's and youths' relationships with adults and peers that contribute to psychological well-being are characterized by interactions that convey genuineness, empathy, unconditional caring, and affirmation (p.8).

Linked to the common values are key concepts such as positive youth development and strength-based perspectives. Importantly, the concept of social-emotional learning (SEL), described in detail later in this chapter, is critical to positive mental health: it is the process by which students develop their own knowledge, skills, and attitudes for positive mental health, healthy relationships, conflict resolution, and more.

The report includes guidelines to incorporate best practices related to positive mental health within a comprehensive school health framework. Organized under the JCSH framework's four pillars, these actions all relate to the goals of student engagement and positive relationships.

Healthy School Policy

- Use discipline policies that are solution-focused, seek to reconnect students to the school community, and are relational in nature.
- Make sure that educators have access to professional development focused on positive mental health perspectives and practices.

Teaching and Learning

- Empower students by understanding and appreciating diversity wherever it occurs in the school community.
- Personalize learning for students by exploring areas of interest, strength, and potential to enhance their engagement in both instruction and relationships.

Social and Physical Environment

- Create accessible meeting spaces where students feel safe and valued in order to develop positive relationships with caring peers and adults.
- Promote awareness and understanding about the mental health needs of students and include these needs in the design of positive learning environments.

Partnerships and Services

- Foster mentorship opportunities for students by partnering and working together with community-based organizations that work with school-aged children and youth.
- Develop positive home–school interactions that support students in achieving their potential.

Bullying Prevention, Conflict Resolution, and Positive Relationships

Having the skills and abilities to build positive relationships is fundamental to a child's healthy growth and development. Many schools are taking a proactive approach to bullying prevention, choosing to focus on healthy, positive relationships. For example, students who have developed the communication skills to explain the difference between bullying and conflict can also identify positive steps for dealing with both.

Building positive relationships takes time and effort; however, there are some essential skills that can help along the way.

- Learn to communicate assertively without being aggressive.
- Active listening skills can help people in conflict put aside their emotions and demonstrate understanding of the other person's point of view.
- Confident body language: making eye contact, holding your head high, squaring your shoulders, and standing or sitting straight all project confidence—be aware of your body language!
- Conflict occurs when there is disagreement between equals. Even if emotions get out of hand and tempers rise, both parties can influence the situation from a position of mutual power. Strategies for successfully managing conflict can include:
    - Negotiating: listen to one another's point of view and discuss what resolution would be best.
    - Compromising: both people agree to sacrifice something to resolve the conflict.
    - Explaining: each person explains their position clearly and calmly without attacking the other person.
    - Asking for intervention: ask an adult (or neutral friend) to listen to both sides and help find a solution.

Bullying differs from conflict in that a bully wants to hurt the other person intentionally. A bully does or says the same things over and over and tries to exert power to intimidate another person. Bullying takes four main forms (or combinations): physical, verbal, social, and electronic. To eliminate or reduce bullying, check out these strategies and many more at www.bullyfreealberta.ca:

- Being bullied? Don't ignore the bully. Stand up for yourself by making eye contact and calmly tell the bully to stop. Ask a friend or an adult to help—keep adults informed about what is happening.
- Bystander? Offer to help the victim and ask them to hang out with you and your friends. Tell the person who is bullying to stop.
- Parent/Guardian? School staff? Check out the facts about bullying and access the many online resources that are available. Talk with children and students about the seriousness of bullying and what we can all do to help eliminate it.

Social-Emotional Learning

Have you ever tried to focus on learning when you are emotionally distressed? Not only is it difficult to focus your thoughts when you are upset about something, but it is also difficult to learn. Students are no different from adults in this respect, which is why social-emotional learning is so important for a healthy school community.

Social-emotional learning (SEL) is a process for learning life skills. These skills apply to each individual, to others, and to relationships. They also help students learn how to work effectively in a variety of contexts. Leaders in health-promoting schools understand that effective learning takes place best in a socially safe and emotionally positive context. Broadly, SEL programs and strategies include self-awareness, self-management, social awareness, relationship skills, and responsible decision making (Collaborative for Academic, Social, and Emotional Learning, 2012).

Since the term "social-emotional learning" was coined, educators and researchers continue to discover the many benefits of SEL. SEL programs have been shown to:

- improve behaviour, resulting in reduced emotional distress, decreased number of disciplinary actions, and improved attendance
- decrease behaviours such as drug use and violence that interfere with learning.
- promote supportive relationships by helping to make best use of cooperative and collaborative learning strategies
- improve learning: engagement is increased, understanding deepens, and students are more likely to develop critical thinking skills and, ultimately, become engaged citizens

If a school is considering adding SEL or improving the delivery of a program already in place, there are several factors to consider. First, SEL should occur in each year of schooling and it should be developmentally appropriate at each level. It is not a "one-time event" but rather a gradual building of awareness, skills, and strategies as a child progresses through school. Second, SEL programs should be used to help shape and define the school's culture and climate. Finally, SEL programs should be structured to develop specific skills within the broad categories described earlier in this section.

Health and Social Justice

Along with recognizing the vital importance of a positive psychosocial environment, health-promoting schools acknowledge the importance of social responsibility. A truly democratic country depends on developing skills and dispositions associated with responsible citizenship supported in a climate of critical thinking. Social responsibility involves developing students who are "socially and critically literate."

In the following article, Dr. Finney Cherian, an associate professor in the Faculty of Education at the University of Windsor, portrays classroom life and the texts he uses to encourage children to explore and understand social justice. This close look at the structure and content of learning provides an opportunity to see how a variety of texts can be activated when health issues are infused into classroom practices.

Clearly, Dr. Cherian is preparing his students to be sensitive to issues related to equity and social justice as a way of being in the world. Additionally, Cherian wants his students to learn how to assert their rights and fulfill their responsibilities in positive ways. For Cherian and his students, learning is about preparing to act with care for self and others in mind.

SUCCESS STORY

Really Teaching Social Justice

By Dr. Finney Cherian

Often discussions focused on the importance of teaching social justice are steeped in abstract philosophical concepts that leave most practitioners uninspired and uninformed as to the best way to teach this topic to their students. What are required are articles limited in "academic jargon" and rich in classroom examples. However, I am not advocating for "goof-proof" curriculum planning, but rather critical explorations of the best ways to encourage our students to ask, "Why are some people advantaged and others disadvantaged, and how am I implicated in the existing social order?" The ensuing discussion is reflective of my journey as an elementary teacher and pre-service teaching instructor in prompting my students at the elementary and university levels to ask such questions.

If our schools are to be places of hope and inspiration, teachers must address the paradox of not only helping each child value themselves, but also helping each child to transcend this self-acceptance and embrace those around them. This article makes no demands for curricular alchemists. Critical teaching practices that attempt to teach concepts like social justice are not grounded in magic; rather, they are embedded in qualities such as empathy, courage, and activism. In creating a classroom committed to social justice, the following ought to be considered: "The process of becoming literate is inseparable from living."

A classroom committed to teaching children about social responsibility must see student collaboration and participation as prerequisites for implementing the goal of teaching social justice. During my years as an elementary teacher serving a poor working-class community, I realized that the phrase "links to home" had to encompass more than letters about student misconduct and newsletters about upcoming bake sales. The phrase had to be broadened to encompass the reality that vibrant classroom communities of learners can exist only if the lives of students and their families are directly linked to the curriculum of the classroom. This bridge is at times extremely difficult for the best of teachers to build, but one that must be attempted by any educator whose teaching goals emerge out of a deep respect for their students (Peterson, 1994).

During the first weeks of school I would often focus activities on gathering as much information as I could about the families of my students (using non-intrusive means). For example, I would provide each child with a large sheet of Bristol board that I cut in the shape of a puzzle piece. I ensured that each puzzle piece interlocked with another Bristol board section. The interlocking pieces symbolized the uniqueness and interconnectedness of our classroom community. I always pointed out to the class that each piece in a jigsaw puzzle helped to create a complete picture. Thus, like a missing piece, the absence or non-involvement of one member of our class would diminish the classroom community and prevent it from being whole.

After students decorated and personalized their pieces, I would staple them to the bulletin boards on the walls of the classroom. On each puzzle piece the students were encouraged to mount family photos. As well, a large zip-locked freezer bag was glued to each piece to hold any special articles that held sentimental value to the student. One year, a student named Sam displayed a pair of his deceased grandfather's dentures. On a descriptive card, he wrote about times when he remembered his grandfather removing his dentures and making him laugh by smiling without any teeth. Another student, Tanya, mounted a pair of her mother's shoes with an explanation that her mother, a single parent, was her hero. Tanya's mother would often tell her that in her mother's absence Tanya would have to "stand in her shoes" and take care of her little brother.

The classroom jigsaw puzzle became a concrete symbol representing the concept of community. Children from diverse economic and ethnic backgrounds and family configurations often found that their lives were more similar than different. The collaborative act of constructing the class jigsaw puzzle helped my elementary students connect with the narrative qualities of their lives, and the lives of others. Being aware of the narrative qualities of others' lives was not only important in motivating them to write about themselves—this awareness was also crucial in helping them develop a reverence for the lives of students with whom they would share learning experiences. Social justice demands that individuals defend the rights of others. Such actions are motivated by a deep-rooted reverence and respect for others. I wanted this sense of respect to manifest itself in students' actions as they advocated for themselves and others whenever their rights, emotional well-being, or safety were at risk.

As the school term progressed, the puzzle pieces were replaced with other displays. However, I continued to encourage my students to draw upon their lived experiences as sources for illuminating publications. I ensured that if the class was studying poetry, they grounded the themes for their poems in the issues that impacted their neighbourhoods and communities. Our first poetry unit of the year often began with neighbourhood walks. I asked students to look for things they were proud of, or things they wanted to change about their neighbourhood. On one such walk we passed Sam's apartment building.

Sam recognized a tenant that he said his neighbours knew to be a constant victim of domestic violence.

Motivated to speak out against domestic violence, Sam later wrote this acrostic poem:

> Apartment Walls Need to Be Thicker
>
> He throws dishes and she screams, "I HATE you!"
>
> Anytime, all the time seems like the right time to fight
>
> They hate each other in the apartment, but kiss in the elevator
>
> Everyone on the floor hears, but no one calls the cops, or cares

In the classroom discussion that followed the reading of Sam's poem, other students shared similar stories. They said that violence was often a part of their lives and they made statements such as:

> "The cops are useless; they never help. My mother says you can't trust them."
>
> "If a man hits a woman, he should go to jail."
>
> "Why can't she just move away? It's her fault for staying with him."

I guided their discussion to uncover the complex variables associated with domestic violence. This discussion provided an opportunity for me to draw students' attention to episodes of violence I had witnessed in the playground during recess and the ways in which students in our classroom often chose to solve problems in a manner similar to Sam's neighbour's behavioural choices.

When students are permitted to connect their lived experiences to their work in class, it helps them to acknowledge the serious and pervasive nature of certain issues in their lives, while helping to guide them to confront and rethink the attitudes they formulate about various social issues. Identifying their own attitudes helps them confront how their beliefs are implicated in finding solutions. For example, Enid Lee (1994: 193) points out that "children should engage in a critique of the roots of inequality in curriculum, school structure, and the larger society—always asking: How are we involved? What can we do?"

The teaching of social justice must be lived through classroom events that are participatory and experiential. Classrooms ought to provoke students to develop their democratic capacities: to question, to challenge, to make real decisions, to collectively solve problems. David Booth (1994) writes: "Learning is a process that begins with the known reality of the children. The teacher helps the learners move beyond, into unknown areas, developing hypotheses about issues and concerns that intrigue them, testing those hypotheses through problem-solving activities and reflecting about the consequences of their actions. By being a part of their learning, by interacting and dialoguing, children come to understand the process of imaginative inquiry" (p.112).

Here is an example of this process in action. When exploring the issue of prejudice through Peter Golenbock's picture book *Teammates*, I decided to use David Booth's and Jonothan Neeland's approaches to writing in role to help students gain perspective on the ugliness of racism. I first read the story to the class and had them write a letter to the main character—Jackie Robinson, the first black player in major league baseball in the United States—describing a time in their lives when they were ridiculed or rejected by others because of their appearance. Many students felt a deep connection to the story, which elicited painful recollections and testimonies concerning racial intolerance.

In our diverse multicultural and multilingual classroom community, there was no shortage of stories about name-calling, except for Andrew. Andrew was the only white student in the class. He proclaimed that no one had ever called him names based on his skin colour: "Mr. Cherian, no one has ever called me a 'nigger' before. I don't know what to write about." I offered Andrew an opportunity to play Jackie Robinson in an improvisation re-enacting one of the most powerful scenes in the book that takes place on a baseball diamond. As Andrew positioned himself on an imaginary first base, other students circled him in role as spectators, calling him names. After debriefing the role play with the class, I asked Andrew to list words or images that came to mind as the others called him names. I then asked him to draw upon ideas from this list during his writing. In his ensuing letter, Andrew described his experience of listening to the story and dramatizing parts of it. Andrew's letter vividly described the anger and sadness he felt as classmates taunted him. In his letter, he wrote, "When the fans were yelling at me, I could not make them stop. I wanted to yell at them, but there were too many of them. They were yelling all at once. The names they called me made me feel like broken glass." Andrew's broken glass analogy was the most powerful way for him to describe the complex perception of emotional fragmentation a person faces when confronted with racism. Andrew's role play allowed him to breach an egocentric perspective and explore subjectivities that were unfamiliar to him. Drama expressed through role play took Andrew from, "I don't know what to write" to, "I felt like broken glass." Booth (1994) eloquently summarizes Andrew's journey as he writes, "Role play allows children to explore the world without risk; to step outside their skin and into the skin of others" (p.279).

It is important to note that the success of this drama lesson was predicated upon the trusting relationship that Andrew and I had developed. This example raises an important question for practitioners and students of drama: How does risk-taking promote learning? In asking this question, we begin to recognize the importance of valuing and making a personal investment in teaching and learning through drama. This does not happen accidentally; it begins at the start of the school year with teachers who intentionally make the elements of a balanced dramatic arts program central to their reading and writing programs.

With respect to the issue of racism, racialized students cannot shed their skin at the end of drama class. However, drama allowed Andrew to see the world through the eyes of others. The issue of social injustice in the form of racism is predicated on differential societal power relations. If equity and equality are to be attained, the responsibility to evoke the greatest societal change rests upon those with the greatest degree of power to do so. As a member of the dominant (white) societal group, Andrew can decide to make such changes. This may appear to be an unfair burden to place on the shoulders of a little boy. However, little boys and girls become men and women who can take these issues beyond our classrooms to other levels of society. An idea can be a dangerous thing. A little white boy like Andrew with a sensitivity toward and disdain for the word "nigger" can confront and challenge the existence of ideologies that limit the life chances and hopes of others. Through the power of classroom drama activities, students from both dominant and subordinate groups can develop a sense of compassion and acceptance for each other. Drama activities can reinforce the reality that if strong actions are not taken against social injustices, these injustices will proliferate. The very preservation of democratic ideals is balanced on this point.

When discussing issues of social justice, it is polite to "talk back." When there is silence, there is often little learning. As a classroom teacher, I have come to believe that all learning must occur on a "sea of talk." The issue of equity and social justice requires both teacher and students to speak out against oppression. They need opportunities to apply and hone the skills they have learned in various curricular areas to explore social-justice issues.

For example, the math concepts of percentage and graphing can become lenses through which students can explore issues related to social equity. Once students learn the rudiments of collecting data and constructing bar graphs, they can refine their skills by answering questions such as, "What percentage of models represented in popular fashion magazines are Black and Asian?" Predictably, when my students surveyed various magazines and constructed bar graphs, they noticed the sparse representation of certain ethnic groups. In my class, such findings formed the content around which the class learned to write letters to the editors of the magazines they surveyed.

Not only did my students learn "proper letter-writing form," but they were also motivated to seek answers to questions such as "Why are there comparatively few Black and Asian models in fashion magazines?" One student named Jordan wrote, "You like the colour of money when I buy your magazine, but no one in it looks like me." Unfortunately, our letters to several editors went unanswered. However, the students and I discussed the possibility that the silence that their letters received may have reflected the discomfort that their questions caused individuals who were unwilling to justify the racial and ethnic inequity evident in their magazines.

To teach social justice is to teach social action. Silence and non-action are the great complements to maintaining social inequities. To this end, students must use their abilities in reading, writing, and mathematics to "talk back" to the existing social order by asking difficult questions. A class committed to embracing social justice encourages students to look for bias in literature. "Reading is not exhausted merely by decoding the written word or written language, but rather anticipated by extending into knowledge of the world. Reading the world precedes reading the word and the subsequent reading of the word cannot dispense with continually reading the world" (Friere, 1983: 139). Freire's sentiments implicitly demand a reconceptualization of the relationship between text and reader. The notion that reading is strictly a private affair unfairly ignores the multiple attachments of social identities and shared experience that constitute the history of the text (via the author) and the history of the reader. Engagement with the text and the world determines not only how others think about us, but also how we think of ourselves. The text, its author, and its audience emerge into discourse and discursive practices that define, organize, and regulate the sense of who they are in relation to others and the physical world (Simon, 1992).

Freire's notion of reading the world and the word defines reading as a private and public enterprise embedded in historical ways of knowing and seeing the world. Language and reality are dynamically interwoven.

The cleavages created between literacy and reality can prove to be a painful location for individuals marginalized by their racial, class, gender, and sexual identities. Words like "nigger," "bitch," and "faggot" are not benign nouns but are symbolic road signs that, when encountered, cause a reader to detour into reliving painful experiences. In response to political pressure, academic institutions have begun to assess certain texts for the appropriateness of their inclusion in educational curriculum. This trend asks whether the anticipation of "reader pain" through circumstances involving specific literary language merits removal of certain texts from classrooms. The notion of a literary canon being challenged by teachers, parents, guardians, and academics advocating for the removal of controversial texts may facilitate detours of historical pain. However, in questioning the intrinsic value of various texts, stakeholders have reduced the debate around text to a duality between good literature and bad literature, while leaving no space to consider the value of subversive text (Simon, 1992).

I have found that examining text that is steeped in bias is necessary in supporting my goal of teaching social justice. For example, *Little Black Sambo* by Helen Bannerman (1889) was extremely useful in guiding discussion about how certain groups such as Blacks have been distorted and villainized throughout history in extremely painful ways. I found it necessary to provoke students into reflection about how certain artistic styles and characterizations propagate stereotypes. When students encountered texts and images that did not affirm who they were, I encouraged them to find images that did provide self-affirmation.

Teaching from a social-justice perspective compels students to learn to become critical consumers, producers, and transformers of text. Thus, educators might consider the following suggestions:

- Help students consider the perspectives and interpretations of the author and the illustrator of a text.
- Students and teachers can examine together a story's context, historical background, depiction of characters, and points of reference in order to detect and analyze bias and stereotyping.
- Examine images and illustrations closely to detect racial, class-related, and gender-based biases and stereotypes.
- Examine the social messaging in resources being used in the classroom to ensure a balance between texts that promote social and cultural information and texts designed to entertain.
- Be attentive to students' reactions and seek out their honest opinions and perspectives. ■

Case Study

By Amanda Stanec

Reema is about to graduate with a Bachelor of Education degree and has accepted a position as a high school health and physical education teacher in a small town. The high school shares a property with the local elementary school. Reema's teaching assignment for her first job placement includes a combination of health, physical education, and social studies. She is nervous about having three content areas to teach during her first year but there is no way she would turn down this position.

During her hiring interview, Reema spoke passionately about her interest in social justice, service learning as an instructional model, and supporting all students' psychosocial development. She was somewhat surprised when the principal called and told her that she was awarded the job over other more experienced teachers.

The principal told Reema that she was selected because the school wants someone on staff who is committed to implementing service learning, as well as someone who is prepared to support other teachers in furthering students' psychosocial development.

1 What challenges are presented in this case study? How significant are they? Do you think you could solve these challenges easily? On your own?
2 Put yourself in Reema's shoes. What immediate steps would you take to decrease or minimize stressful feelings? Why did you choose these steps? Can a minimal level of stress be an asset?
3 What personal strengths (such as leadership and organizational skills and work experience) would you bring to help navigate these challenges? Why do you think these strengths would be helpful? Have you applied them in other instances in which they have served you well? If so, what results did you achieve?
4 If you were Reema, how would you combine service learning and psychosocial development with health education and social studies? Consider what a social-justice approach might look like using these three subjects and accessing both school and community resources.
5 What personal health strategies would you encourage Reema to adopt in order to have the best year possible? How might she be a role model for both students and teachers without being "preachy"?

It's Your Turn

1 Develop short-term and long-term goals, as well as performance measures to track progress, to apply content from this chapter to your current pre-service teacher setting or employment setting.

2 Create an assessment strategy to determine the effectiveness of the goals presented in question 1.

✓ Action Checklist

Individual	Suggested Follow-up
Pre-service Teacher	❑ During practicum placements, find ways to use different instructional models, such as service learning, in several content areas. ❑ Whenever possible, find ways to support students' psychosocial development in your lesson plans; share your ideas with peers and ask for their feedback.
Health and Physical Education Teacher	❑ Collaborate closely with classroom teachers in your school to familiarize yourselves with ways to integrate learning while maintaining HPE outcomes as your highest priority. ❑ Meet with a service learning coordinator in your school district to determine ways to incorporate successful service learning programs. ❑ Plan ways to implement service learning as an instructional model in health education. ❑ Collaborate with other content-area teachers to implement service-learning programs.
Administrator	❑ Ensure that new professionals' health and previous experience are considered when assigning teaching loads and courses. ❑ Implement mentoring programs so that teachers who teach more than two content areas receive support.
Parent / Guardian	❑ Ask school administrators if service learning is used as an instructional model in their school and let them know you believe service learning is a great option for character education along with content knowledge. ❑ Find ways to support your school in initiating, planning, and implementing service-learning programs.

Chapter 5 Summary

This chapter highlights the pivotal role that schools can play in creating a positive social and emotional environment for teaching and learning. A health-promoting school recognizes the importance of fostering important psychosocial constructs such as quality of life, self-esteem, and personal and social responsibility not only within the school, but in the wider community as well. Health-promoting schools help prepare students to deal with life issues that are relevant and representative of the world in which they live. Such schools also have the potential to provide opportunities for students and the entire school community to become agents for social change. As Dr. Finney Cherian reminds us, with knowledge comes responsibility. It is not enough to teach our students about injustices—it is equally important to equip them with the skills to enact change. Can someone "live the good life" when others around them are suffering? Can someone "feel good about themselves" when others are excluded and marginalized? Health cannot simply be viewed through the eye of the beholder. Rather, care for self must also encompass care for others. Health-promoting schools offer that opportunity, but insist at the same time on everyone's responsibilities to help enhance the health and well-being of all members of the school community.

Questions for Reflection

1 What are the characteristics of a school environment that is supportive of mental health? What are some warning signs that might indicate that a student is dealing with a mental health issue? What are some ways in which a teacher might support that student?

2 Identify some important civil rights in a school setting (e.g., the right to attend school without being made fun of; the right to not be afraid; the right to express your ideas freely). Then identify your responsibilities in ensuring that your civil rights and those of others are upheld.

3 Should certain civil rights be withdrawn from those who have abused the civil rights of others? Justify your answer.

4 Identify different forms of government and use a chart to compare their features. Based on this comparison, what would be an ideal form of government for a model classroom structure and how would it function?

5 List five ideal elements of classroom culture that resonate with your own beliefs about a healthy learning environment. Beside each element, write several steps that you can take to model, promote, and encourage these conditions. How could students become involved in a process designed to improve classroom culture?

6 A teacher decided to set up a "Sports Garden" in his classroom. He invited students to bring old running shoes and worn-out tennis and soccer balls to school. Together they filled each item with potting soil and planted seedlings. Each "shoe-garden," "tennis-ball garden," and "soccer-ball garden" had a story to tell: about its origin, plant care requirements, what it added to the classroom environment, and so on. What is "healthy" about this project?

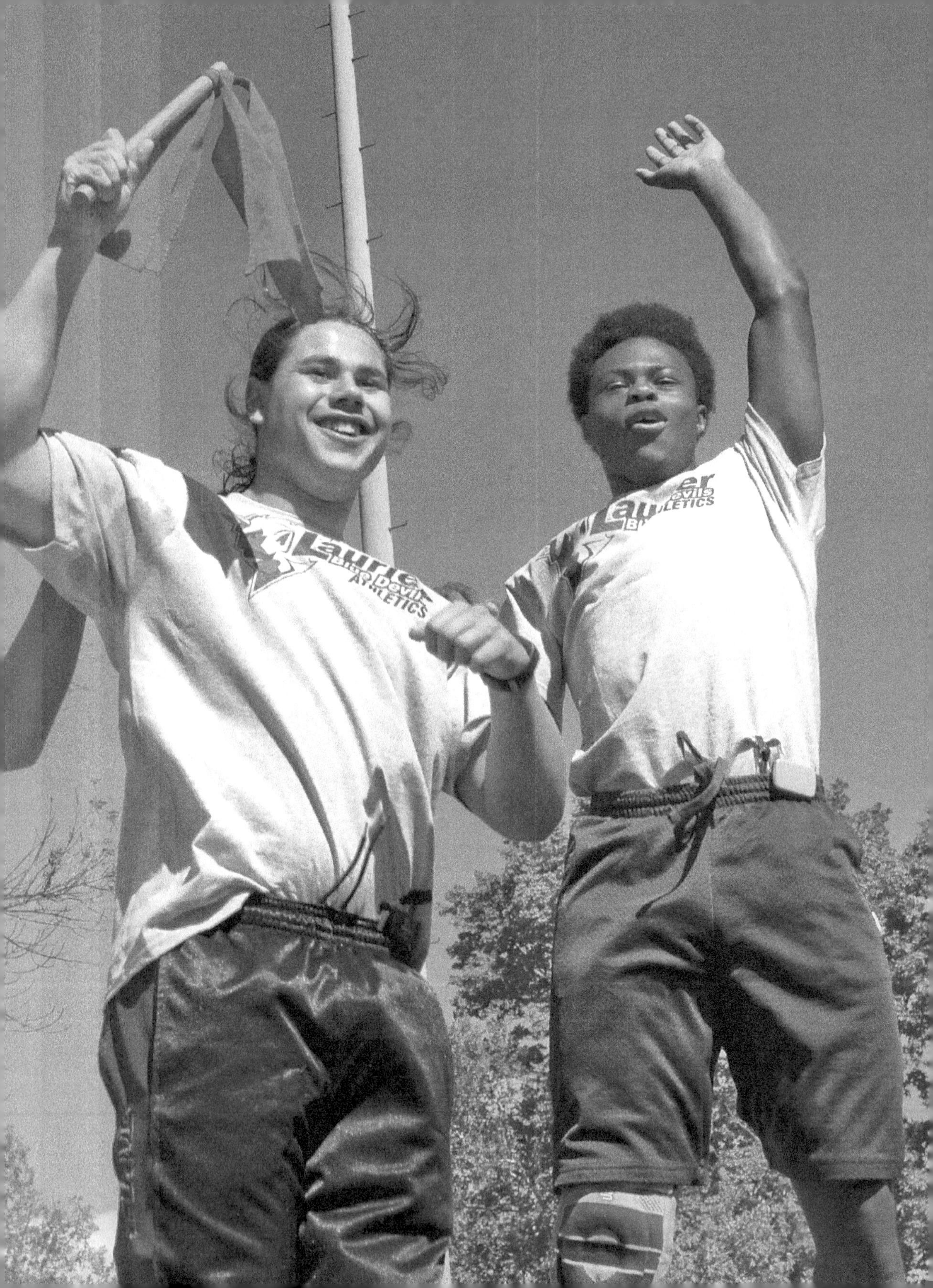
Laurier

6

Social Supports and Healthy Schools

Working together to build resilience

It takes a village to raise a child and it takes a village to educate a student. Responsibility for student learning does not fall entirely on schools. It is an obligation shared with families and the wider community. The degree to which partners in education work together determines whether students' opportunities and choices for healthy living are optimized. Thus, everyone other than teachers who has a vested interest in students (including parents and guardians, school boards, post-secondary institutions, and national and provincial organizations) need to do their part in creating and maintaining health-promoting schools.

Parents, guardians, or other family members can volunteer to help manage extra-curricular programs and clubs. Older students can lead playground activities for younger students. Schools can invite local sports clubs, recreation centres, and public health units to give program demonstrations or host participatory events to raise students' awareness of community-based activities offered outside school hours and during school breaks. At the post-secondary level, university and college professors can encourage their students to volunteer in a local healthy schools program or collaborate with local partners to explore funding opportunities to implement and evaluate initiatives within a healthy school. The key is to work together as a school community toward a common goal of providing opportunities for students to develop the skills, knowledge, and attitudes to lead healthy lives (Mandigo, 2002).

***It is essential to identify and involve concerned partners in the development and implementation of policies and programs promoting physical activity at all levels, especially those targeting school-age children and young people. —* (WHO, 2000, p. 12).**

Without social supports in place, students cannot thrive. A health-promoting school recognizes that students need direct support as well as access to resources in the wider community. In essence, the school becomes a hub connecting students to the social networks they need to live healthy, active lives. A school-based peer mentor program to facilitate social acceptance or cultural awareness is an example of **direct support**. **Indirect support** is offered through school-linked initiatives that give students access to additional resources, such as community recreation programs or local nutrition programs to help control diabetes. Whatever the need or the issue, a healthy school is where students find support and guidance in making healthy choices and decisions.

This chapter serves two purposes. First, it highlights people, organizations, and services that can directly and indirectly impact students' health by forging partnerships with schools. Second, it examines ways in which social supports can maximize the health and well-being of students in a healthy school community.

Four Key Factors Underpinning Social Supports for Students (The Four Fs)

Many evidence-based strategies and programs are available to strengthen the relationships and partnerships upon which health-promoting schools depend for social supports. Of the various factors that underpin development and maintenance of effective social supports for students, four are key: friends, family, finances, and a sense of belonging or "fitting in" as a valued participant in the daily interactions that take place within the school community.

- Friends. In terms of the dimensions of health related to conditions and opportunities for learning, there is a convergence of two domains: health and education. Children and youth who feel disconnected, alienated, and lonely cannot learn optimally. When asked what makes life good for them and the people they care about, students most frequently respond "friends." Clearly, the need for affiliation, acceptance, belonging, and inclusion is crucial to each child's social and mental health. School may be the one place where children can play safely with peers, laugh, tell stories, and confide in and comfort others.

  A clear example of the power of peer relationships for children is the FRIENDS program in British Columbia. Operated by the provincial health care system, this free, multi-level program is designed to help children not only learn to establish and maintain quality relationships but also reduce anxiety and build resiliency. FRIENDS aligns with the core competencies of the British Columbia curriculum, teaching specific skills related to social-emotional learning: self-management, self-awareness, social awareness, relationship skills, and responsible decision making. It also promotes the qualities and capabilities that the Dalai Lama Center for Peace and Education describes as essential for a child's "heart-mind well-being":

  - gets along with others
  - is compassionate and kind
  - solves problems peacefully
  - is secure and calm
  - is alert and engaged

- Family. By nurturing their children physically and emotionally, families play a critical role in their children's journey to adopt a healthy lifestyle. Families come in many forms. In some cases, a primary caregiver (e.g., mother, father, guardian, or grandparent) may be the sole influence. In some extended families, members other than primary caregivers (such as an aunt, uncle, elder, sibling, or cousin) may play a more influential role. Regardless, education, particularly health education, is a shared responsibility that cannot simply be left to the teacher and the school. In order for students to apply and integrate health concepts into their daily lives, they need the support of all members of their family. From a physical activity perspective, here are three ways to encourage families to support healthy active living:
- Communication channels. Provide quality information to families about the benefits of physical activity and locally based opportunities to be active together. Ideas include publishing a regular school newsletter section devoted to getting families moving together, connecting families to activities their children are learning in physical education, placing a dedicated bulletin board in a high-traffic area of the school, encouraging active transport for families (see Chapter 4), and posting a page dedicated to family activities and outings on the school website.
- Community events and get-togethers. Consider using the school as a social and recreational hub where community members can gather. Invite families to engage in events such as:
  - Family triathlon: Set up a local triathlon (or duathlon if you do not have access to a pool) for the community and encourage families to swim, bike, and run as they complete the course together.
  - Family dance party: After students learn a variety of dances in physical education class, invite families to a "barn dance"-style event (consider connecting the dance with the social studies curriculum). Consider the diverse cultures in your community and invite demonstrations and instruction in various dance styles for community members.
  - Family fitness centre: Consider developing a space that can be used by students and staff during the day and by community members during the evening (supervised by appropriate personnel). Apply for grants to help cover equipment and renovation costs.
- School-based opportunities. Energize some of the routine school events for parents such as:
  - Parent-teacher interviews: Provide activity stations in the gym or in an open classroom so that children can participate with their parents between interviews.
  - Open houses: Provide a physical education station run by current students for prospective students and their families.
  - Add large-group energizers to parent-oriented assemblies, for example, chair yoga or ice-breaking activities that help relax participants.
  - Include some physical activity as part of special school events such as volunteer teas, grandparents' day, holiday concerts, and awards ceremonies.

- Finances—Meeting the needs of a variety of learners. Children's lives outside school cannot be overlooked. The cultures and communities in which young people grow up influence their growth and development, thus impacting their learning and their health. Children and youth may experience a variety of difficulties that teachers need to take into account. Robert Marzano's *Building Background Knowledge for Academic Achievement* (2004) examines the consequences of poverty on children's learning, for example. Children living in poverty experience difficulties that present enormous challenges to their learning process. It is important to be aware of the constraints that children living in poverty and near poverty must cope with in order to succeed as learners. A child in a low-income situation is less likely to have access to print and technology resources or to have money to buy project materials such as markers and poster paper. Additionally, some children receive no encouragement at home to pursue academic success. To compound the problem, in some friendship groups academic achievement is ridiculed. Doing well in school means students have conformed or given in to authority. Teachers need to understand these factors in order to find ways for all students to learn and be healthy.

  Children and youth in low-income households often live with the daily anxiety of not knowing whether there will be food to eat or whether a parent's job is secure. Children worry about their parents' happiness. A parent who is discouraged and hurt shares those disappointments with the family. As a parent's mental health declines, substance use and problems related to violence may result, making matters even worse. For many children living in poverty, school is a refuge, offering stability, consistency, and unconditional acceptance. For these children especially, school activities can make a significant positive difference to their health and well-being. Recognizing these difficulties means educators may need to set aside curriculum concerns temporarily and interact with the child as a unique individual with unique emotional and pragmatic needs requiring immediate attention. As the expression goes, "You need to take care of Maslow before you can address Bloom" (referring to Maslow's hierarchy of needs and Bloom's taxonomy).
- Fitting in—Fostering a sense of connectedness. Children and youth who feel that they are a valuable part of their school community and that the community cares about them are less likely to get into trouble. They also have higher levels of emotional well-being. Fitting in or belonging at school is often called *school connectedness.* Interactions with adults and peers, curricular and extra-curricular activities, school-board policies, and everyday practices all affect the level of connectedness a child feels at school. Students who feel that they belong and are connected to others most likely experience some or all of the following:
  - high level of teacher support and care for individual students
  - good friends at school
  - attentiveness to current and future academic performance
  - school discipline policies that are fair and efficient
  - participation in extra-curricular activities

Benefits of school connectedness can be broadly divided into three categories:

- Academic achievement. Connected students are more likely to attend school regularly, pay attention to their grades, and pursue post-secondary education.
- Reduction of high-risk behaviours. Students who feel a sense of belonging to the school community are less likely to be involved in high-risk behaviours such as smoking, alcohol and substance misuse, early sexual activity, drinking and driving, suicide attempts, and weapon-related violence.
- Mental well-being. Connected students are less likely to experience emotional distress or abuse, can handle stress effectively, and are more resilient—that is, they have the ability to bounce back from duress.

It is important to talk with children and youth about how connected they feel at school and about the factors that influence their sense of connectedness. The JCSH stresses:

> Evidence points to the importance of building the strongest possible sense of community around the student. Connectedness with family, school, and community are central protective factors. Problems such as substance use that arise in many schools should never be seen as an isolated negative issue but within the context of a network of relationships that values the individual. Schools can create the conditions and structures that enable such relationships to be built and maintained. Teachers who understand that education is more than imparting information and invest in building mentoring relationships can play a turnaround role for many students. Non-teaching school professionals (e.g., counsellors, administrative and janitorial staff) can also provide mentoring relationships to students who may be at risk of disconnecting from school. (JCSH, 2009)

Building Parent Engagement: A Vital Social Support

Meaningful parental/guardian involvement is essential in creating and sustaining a healthy school community. In an article published in *Education Canada* in 2013, Lorna Costantini shares a wealth of information about how school communities can involve parents most effectively. Here is a summary of what Costantini recommends:

> First, ask for input. This simple step is often neglected in the rush to get things done. Invite two-way dialogue using a variety of media and be transparent about processes and decisions. Second, lead by example. Be a believer in the fact that parent engagement works and improves learning for kids. Third, recognize that there are limiting factors that may interfere with the level of interaction parents can have with schools. These limitations include time, language barriers, cultural barriers, and religious beliefs. Be creative and reach out to those whose voices may not be heard regularly. Fourth, make an effort to help parents understand what happens on a day-to-day basis at the school. Refrain from using "edu-speak" and jargon—it can be confusing and even humiliating for those who do not understand terms that educators may take for granted. Use a variety of methods and media to provide an accurate portrayal of your school or your class.

> Finally, allow parent leaders (they are there already!) to become allies and to step forward to support the policies, programs, and vision of the school. Recognize that these leaders can be a powerful force for good. Communicate with them frequently and help them to feel a sense of ownership with respect to the school and the resources and opportunities that the school community can provide to students. (Costantini, 2013)

Partnering with Families and Communities: The Epstein Model

A well-organized program of family and community partnerships yields many benefits for schools and their students. What is the difference between a professional learning community and a school learning community? *A professional learning community* emphasizes teamwork among principals, teachers, and staff to identify school goals, improve curriculum and instruction, reduce teachers' isolation, assess student progress, and increase the effectiveness of school programs. Professional teamwork is important: it can greatly improve teaching, instruction, and professional relationships in a school. However, it falls short of producing a true community of learners. In contrast, a *school learning community* includes educators, students, parents, guardians, and community partners who work together to improve the school and enhance students' learning opportunities.

One component of a school learning community is an organized program of school, family, and community partnerships with activities linked to school goals. Research and fieldwork show that such programs improve schools, strengthen families, invigorate community support, and increase student achievement and success (Epstein, 2002; Henderson & Mapp. 2002; Sheldon, 2003). Dr. Joyce Epstein, a professor at Johns Hopkins University, has spent several decades researching parental involvement in schools. Her framework for developing partnerships (known as the Epstein Model) describes six clear ways to involve parents (Eptein & Salinas, 2004).

1 **Help parents parent.** By providing information, local connections, and resources on topics such as healthy eating, physical activity, and mental well-being, schools can help parents do their jobs better.

2 **Communicate broadly and frequently.** As discussed earlier, there are many ways for schools to communicate effectively with parents about healthy active living. It is important that parents be kept informed about their children's academic progress, school events, and opportunities to get involved with the school.

3 **Share opportunities to volunteer.** Let parents know that their volunteer contributions are appreciated and supported. Communicate ways for parents to volunteer that do not always involve them coming to the school.

4 **Encourage home learning.** Connect what is learned at school to activities that families can do at home. For example, a social studies class might choose a "dinner table topic" each week for families to discuss on the weekend as they share a meal together. Both the conversation and the act of sharing a meal together are healthy and educational!

5 **Involve parents in school decisions.** Whether it is a graduation celebration, planning a school garden, or developing a healthy food policy—invite parents to help make key decisions about important matters.

6 **Invite community collaboration.** Connect parents to local partners, resources, and services. Invite partners into the school and to parent meetings to share strategies and publicize campaigns or programs related to healthy active living.

For more on the Epstein Model, see "The School, Family, and Community Partnerships: Your handbook for action" (Epstein, et al., 2002) or "Partnering with Families and Communities"(Epstein and Salinas, 2004).

Examples of Successful School–Family–Community Collaboration

A school community works with many partners to increase students' learning opportunities and experiences. Activities to enrich students' skills and talents may be conducted during lunch, after school, and at other times by school, family, and community partners (Sanders, 2001; Sanders & Harvey, 2002). For example, teachers in the middle grades at Good Shepherd School in Peace River, Alberta, asked community instructors in tai chi, tae kwon do, and hip-hop dance to volunteer their time to conduct fitness classes for students during the lunch hour. This program, known as Try It at Lunch, increased activity levels and engagement for many students and increased interest in these community programs after school and on weekends.

Manitoba Education and Training has modelled its Community Schools Partnership Initiative (CSPI) on approaches that the neighbouring province of Saskatchewan adopted to establish "community schools." In Saskatchewan, SchoolPlus is a framework that provides a comprehensive range of supports and approaches to meet the diverse needs of children, youth, and their families. It also provides a basis for schools to develop unique responses to meet specific objectives. Like SchoolPlus, Manitoba's CSPI is designed to help schools in low socio-economic communities enhance education outcomes by developing and strengthening partnerships. CSPI is a long-term effort to encourage families, organizations, and schools to work together to improve students' success and strengthen communities. Schools are a traditional meeting place for community residents and the community school concept builds on that relationship. Children are better able to achieve their educational and developmental potential when there is a working relationship among family, teachers, local service agencies, and the general community.

By strengthening the community schools concept in the province, Manitoba Education and Training continues efforts to improve student learning, strengthen families, and build healthier communities. Parents, community, students, and service delivery agencies can come together in the community school's welcoming environment, nurturing a greater sense of interdependence and community spirit. These schools provide gathering places for adults and children to enjoy educational, social, cultural, and recreational activities. Community schools not only provide supports for school-aged children. Programs may meet the needs of pre-school children, youth, and adults as well. They may be sponsored by partnerships of parents, government, the education community, or other interested partners. They may be based on the specific needs of a whole community, such as after-school programs or community health care, and marshal the resources to meet these needs. A successful community school will assist students and families in the following ways:

- children and youth will start their school days alert and healthy with their basic needs met
- school staff can draw on the community's resources to help students succeed academically and socially
- the health, recreational, cultural, and social services that students need are provided on-site at the school
- parents and community partners provide support to the school and its activities
- the entire community functions as a resource centre to strengthen schools and the community as a whole

Wapanohk-Eastwood Community School in Thompson, Manitoba introduced one of the first community school initiatives. Surveys of parents and students showed that most were very satisfied with the results. The project has led to fewer behavioural problems among students, stronger participation rates of students in school cultural activities, and more awareness among parents about the importance of school success.

Community schools build relationships that contribute to community identity and a neighbourhood's sense of commitment and caring. Manitoba Education and Training and its partners are working to organize interested funders, develop a pool of resources to promote the bridging of service delivery systems, and organize leadership training programs for educators, human service providers, parents, guardians, and community residents through the Community Schools Partnership Initiative.

In Ontario, The Learning Partnership has completed a three-year project called FACES (Family and Community Engagement Strategy). The goal has been to extend and enrich its Welcome to Kindergarten program and provide further community/school-based support for families of young children. With funding from the Ontario Trillium Foundation, the FACES project has been implemented in three Ontario communities: Cornwall, Durham, and Sudbury. The FACES projects broaden and deepen the impact of the Welcome to Kindergarten program by providing enhanced support for:

- family-focused follow-up and enrichment sessions as needed to further nurturing of community-coordinated activities
- more dynamic community partner involvement
- identification of early learning resources available to both teachers and parents

SUCCESS STORY

Six Nations Reserve Healthy Schools Project

By June Sowden (Six Nations Reserve) and Nancy Francis (Brock University)

These two examples demonstrate the vital importance of respect for diversity and celebrations of culture within a healthy school community.

Cultural Days

Students at Oliver M. Smith Kawenni:io Elementary School in Ohsweken, Ontario, always enjoy cultural days. One day each month, students and teachers experience traditional teaching from community experts and respected community elders.

The topic one day was traditional hunting and bread making. As the boys filed into the gym, you could see excitement and eagerness in their faces. Along one wall, four archery targets were set up waiting for arrows to be fired at them.

Teacher Jeremy Green had no problem acquiring the attention of these youngsters. They were all very keen to learn. Everyone sat quietly and listened attentively as Mr. Green explained the features and complexities of the bow and arrow. The boys would learn to respect the intricacies of using a bow and arrow and soon become adept at hitting a target. The class learned that hunting with either a bow and arrow, crossbow, or firearm is still a modern-day custom of many Indigenous people, as well as non-Indigenous people, in Canada, and that it is a lifestyle that promotes healthy living.

Meanwhile, elders were teaching the girls the art of traditional bread making. The girls learned that the dough must be mixed just right; otherwise their bread would come out as hard as hockey pucks. Kneading the dough too much would also result in the same outcome.

Like almost everything else in this world, the girls learned that the secret to good bread making only comes with years of practice!

Learning to Smoke Dance

There was hustle and bustle on the day of the "Learn to Smoke Dance" demonstration at Jamieson Elementary School, also in Ohsweken, Ontario. Inside the gym, students and curious parents lined the walls, not sure what to expect.

The smoke dancers arrived and changed into their traditional Iroquoian regalia and waited for Cam Hill (a local member of the Six Nations community and a popular singer) to arrive with his drum and distinctive voice. No microphone was necessary to project Cam's big voice as he sang. The beating of the drum ignited the dancers' feet.

After a few demonstrations from the experts, everyone was invited to try smoke dancing. Spectators became participants, so that they could appreciate the physical capabilities of the smoke dance competitors they had so often seen at powwows. (At competitions, the drumbeat is very rapid and dancers sometimes must perform continuously through four or five songs to test their athletic ability.)

At the end of the smoke dance demonstration, a sort of "time warp" took place. Students and spectators were invited to try out "Dance, Dance, Revolution," a Nintendo Wii game. The expert smoke dancers became students of the students, as it was now their turn to learn to dance as part of a video game.

This Cultural Day at Oliver M. Smith Kawenni:io Elementary School proved to be an eventful and successful experience for everyone! ■

Acknowledgments

This work was supported through a donation from the Heart and Stroke Foundation of Ontario. Members of the Drumming Hearts Committee include: Lois Bomberry, June Sowden, and Kim Davey of Six Nations Reserve; Bethany Letto of the Heart and Stroke Foundation; and Lyndsey Matsumura (student) and Nancy Francis of Brock University. Nia:weh (thank you) to everyone who made this initiative successful!

Social Supports for At-Risk Students and Their Families

In a two-and-a-half-year study, Hart and Risley (1995) observed interactions between parents and 42 children initially aged two and under. The levels of family wealth ranged from poverty to affluence. For research purposes, Hart and Risley categorized the families into three groups: welfare families, working-class families, and professional families. Major findings of the study (as cited in Marzano, 2004) included:

- The amount of attention and love shown to children had nothing to do with family income.
- Children in families on welfare frequently felt isolated, sometimes because of the dangers associated with playing in their neighbourhood.
- Welfare parents were particularly persistent in ensuring that their children were happy, safe, healthy, and did well in school.
- Children in welfare families were exposed to a fraction of the language that children in working-class and professional families were exposed to.
- Children in welfare families received fewer affirmation statements (e.g., keep trying, you can do it) and more prohibitive statements than those from non-welfare homes.

Schools can help children in vulnerable families, not by replacing parental support but by supplementing it. In schools, statements of affirmation appear in many forms. Bulletin boards, wall murals, and classroom displays are public sites designed to exhibit and celebrate students' works individually and collectively. These displays are more than decorations. They make a statement about the learning, values, and achievements of students. A character wall, for instance, might include examples of student perseverance across a range of activities such as athletic training, working through a science experiment, practising for a concert, or applying science and mathematics concepts and skills to a real-life problem such as erosion control.

Be alert to the needs of your less advantaged students! Cumulatively, lower household income can render children and families more vulnerable to:

- addiction to alcohol, prescription medications, and tobacco
- mental health disorders such as depression, grief, loneliness, and anorexia
- visual and hearing impairments or disorders
- hunger: malnourished, overfed but undernourished, eating disorders
- low self-esteem
- neglect by a parent/guardian
- racism
- a lack of understanding about the importance of supporting high school completion and pathways to post-secondary study (college, trades, or university)

The Families and Schools Together (FAST) Intervention Program

FAST is an award-winning multifamily group intervention program designed to strengthen protective factors for children, empower parents to be primary risk-prevention agents, and build supportive parent-to-parent groups. It brings parents, children, teachers, and the wider community together to help ensure children get the social support they need to fulfill their potential at school—and in life. Both affluent and low-income families struggle with the same issues concerning how to raise a child successfully. Many parents feel alone, too busy to connect with their children, and lacking in support from other adults. Using parent-professional collaborative teams, the FAST program systematically reaches out to entire families and organizes multifamily groups to increase parent involvement with at-risk youth. Developed in 1987 by Dr. Lynn McDonald of Family Service (a non-profit, family counselling agency in Madison, Wisconsin), FAST has been especially successful at involving low-income, stressed, and isolated parents.

With its emphasis on bringing together *local* support resources to build protective factors around children, FAST has been introduced successfully in 18 countries, including Canada. For example, both the Calgary Board of Education and the Calgary Catholic Board of Education run a successful FAST program. By building supportive relationships within families and across communities, FAST helps improve children's engagement in learning and can have a significant positive impact on their life chances and well-being. FAST supports families by:

- helping children improve their skills in reading, writing, and math—as well as encouraging pro-social behaviour and a positive attitude to school and learning
- helping parents become more involved in their child's education, so they can support learning and development at home
- encouraging stronger bonds between parents and their child, their child's school, other parents, and the wider community

The specific program goals for FAST are:

1. Enhance family functioning
    - Strengthen the parent-child relationship in specific, focused ways.
    - Empower the parents to be the primary prevention agents for their children.
2. Prevent the child from experiencing school failure
    - Improve the child's short- and long-term behaviour and performance in school.
    - Empower the parents to be partners in the educational process.
    - Increase the child's and family's feelings of affiliation with their school.
3. Prevent substance abuse by the child and family
    - Increase the family's knowledge and awareness of substance abuse and the impact of substance abuse on child development.
    - Link the family to appropriate assessment and treatment services, as needed.

4. Reduce the stress that parents and children experience from daily life situations
    - Develop an on-going support group for parents of at-risk children.
    - Link the family to appropriate community resources and services, as needed.
    - Build the self-esteem of each family member.

Research has shown that after taking part in the FAST program, children are happier at home and at school and are more engaged in learning. Parent-child bonds improve, family conflicts decrease, parents' involvement in school increases, and social support networks develop between parents. Between 2009 and 2015, nearly 12 thousand families took part in the FAST program in the United Kingdom. Those who took part during the 2013–2014 school year reported that children's behavioural problems decreased by 26%, family conflicts dropped by 24%, and 74% of parents felt more able to support their child in their education.

In summary, the FAST prevention and early intervention program helps children succeed by empowering parents, connecting families, improving the school climate, and strengthening community engagement. For more than 30 years, FAST has achieved consistent positive outcomes in thousands of settings around the world—across ethnicities, cultures, languages, and socio-economic class. This consistency is the result of running each FAST program as it was designed, according to evidence-based practices proven to change children's lives for the better.

Substance Use in Canadian Schools (JCSH)

High-risk youth often come from socially or economically marginalized groups or experience personal factors that contribute to real or perceived disconnection. These students require greater levels of support. Universal education programs lack sufficient focus or intensity to address their needs. Responding effectively to high-risk youth involves helping them develop strong linkages within the school environment. This means helping them develop social and emotional competence and ensuring that the school culture supports their engagement.

A resource developed by the JCSH, *Responding to the Needs of Higher Risk Youth: A Knowledge Kit for Counsellors and Health Workers* (2009), provides a framework, a summary of the evidence, and tools to support school professionals in developing a continuum of programs and services targeted to these students. Consistency between school and community is important. This does not mean, however, that the school should simply reflect community norms and common beliefs. The school has a role in influencing the community as well. At the same time, careful consideration of community values and norms will help in developing effective and contextually relevant policy and educational strategies. Strong school-family-community partnerships can contribute to this multi-directional flow and to the effectiveness of educational efforts at school.

The following table lists various risk factors and protective factors to consider in determining how a school community can support children and youth who are at risk.

Supporting High-Risk Children and Youth: Risk Factors and Protective Factors

	Risk Factors	Protective Factors
Community	• economic disadvantage • social or cultural discrimination or isolation • availability of substances and high tolerance for use	• opportunities for meaningful participation in community groups and activities • involvement with adult mentors and role models
Family	• low parental expectations • tolerant parental attitudes toward teen alcohol/substance use • parental mental illness or substance use problems	• family nurturance and attachment • high level of participation with adults
Peer	• peer rejection • member of deviant peer group	• member of pro-social peer group
School	• poor attachment to school • poor school performance • difficulty at transition points (e.g., entering school, transition to secondary school)	• caring relationships within the school community • high but achievable expectations
Individual	• temperament (sensation seeking, poor impulse control) • high levels of aggression • early regular substance use	• ability to genuinely experience emotions and assert needs • sense of agency and optimism • good literacy and capacity for problem solving

The Impact of Social Supports on Students' Ability to Thrive

Teachers are not social workers, nurses, or police officers. However, in instances when a child needs special services, a teacher may take on a primary role to help children and families access the services and support they need.

In a health-promoting school, access to services should be linked directly to learning and school improvement programs. In many parts of the world, public health providers base many of their health services in the school, offering students access to "one-stop shopping" for a wide range of services and supports. In Finland, for example, doctors and dentists have set up clinics in schools. In the United Kingdom, local coaches are invited to physical education classes to demonstrate and talk about sporting opportunities in the community. In a school near Toronto, hallways are referred to as streets. Corridors running from the central plaza are pathways to offices that offer student counselling, employment services, a health nurse's station, and housing services. The school has become a genuine hub for the delivery of a wide range of social, academic, and health-related services.

Teachers can help students overcome some of the psychosocial barriers associated with service access. Role playing can be especially effective, providing important opportunities for students to understand how the various health and social service systems work, how to care for self and others, how to rehearse their roles, and how to script questions and concerns. Many situations can invite role playing:

- meeting with a counsellor or nurse to talk about issues related to sexual health and safety
- managing relationship issues such as emotional or physical abuse
- having to leave home
- coping with an alcoholic parent
- resolving conflict with a teacher
- applying for a job

When business downsizing and company layoffs occur in a community, schools can host discussions about how students can cope with their own and their parents' feelings of insecurity. The school that cares for students' lives beyond school attendance brings these concerns into focus.

Consider this real-world example of how social supports can help students deal with situational challenges that might otherwise impede learning and a sense of connectedness to the school community:

In a school located near a prison, the student population was in constant flux. Students might attend for a few months and then leave to attend another school in another part of the province. The staff and students wanted to ensure that each new student and their family would be welcomed regardless of length of stay, circumstances, and needs. They formed a welcome team composed of students, teachers, community health professionals, and parents and guardians. Within a few days of a new student's arrival, the student was on a house league team, had signed out a library book, had received free bus tickets and passes to the local YMCA, and was enrolled in a breakfast program at school. Each student's family met with a teacher to tour the school and learn about community services and supports, including health clinics, temporary employment services, child care services, sports programs, and adult learning programs. As well, a local service club installed a washer and dryer at the school. Parents were welcome to do laundry while sitting with their child to read and enjoy learning together. When a child left the school, the student was given a scrapbook containing completed work and photographs of the school and classmates. At this school, it was made very clear that all children and their families deserve to be treated with respect, dignity, and compassion.

Health as a Way to Understand Culture

Often, health as a course of study focuses on clinical interpretations of food and eating, covering subjects such as food groups, nutrient content, and food intake. Learning outcomes set by education departments in each province and territory predetermine what students are expected to know and be able to do. However, when viewed under the banner of a health-performing school, a deeper respect for and understanding of cultural differences can occur. For example, understanding food and eating can also help students better understand the uniqueness and traditions of various cultures. From a cultural perspective, students would be encouraged to examine food preparation, food preservation, and the role of food and eating in a society. How is food a part of the way we socialize and celebrate special occasions? How is food a part of our relationships—at home, in the community, among friends?

Nelson's story as told by Andy:

On the island of Barbuda off the coast of Antigua, I spent an afternoon with Nelson, a local islander. He told me that when he was a boy they caught fish with a stick fashioned into a spear. He said in those days the fish didn't know about people that much and so were not afraid when he and his friends entered the water. They were careful not to disturb this friendly relationship. In some areas where large numbers of fish were harvested, the fish had learned to scatter when people were in the water. Nelson and his friends waited until most fish swam away, leaving one or two behind. These were the ones they caught and cooked over the open fires with plenty of fresh herbs and butter.

From a health perspective, stories such as this offer teachings about culture and traditions. In turn, this learning creates a social environment that is respectful of diverse backgrounds and experiences. Nelson's story is more than a lesson about fishing in a particular country. At a deeper level, it can be used to teach students about concepts such as the complex interaction between humans and their environment, the importance of patience and hard work, and the benefits of cooperation and friendship.

Forging Family-School Partnerships with Newcomer Families

Canada is largely a nation of immigrants. People from diverse cultures, languages, religions, and traditions come to Canada to build new futures, start afresh, and in some cases rebuild broken lives. Immigrants—especially refugees—have unique needs but can also offer diverse perspectives and rich learning to a healthy school community. In an article titled "Designing and Implementing School, Family, and Community Collaboration Programs in Quebec, Canada," Rollande Deslandes (2006) states, "Studies have confirmed that children's education is very important to immigrant parents." Deslandes describes several factors unique to immigrant parents as they strive to adapt to a new country and help their children to succeed:

- Immigrant parents may withdraw if they feel their interactions with their own children are viewed negatively (due to cultural or religious differences).
- Immigrant parents often are forced to take insecure jobs, which means less flexibility and time to attend school functions.
- The level of involvement and engagement of immigrant parents is affected by the degree of cultural and linguistic differences between Canada and their former country.
- Immigrant parents are faced with culture shock stemming from having to bridge different school systems, and from changing roles as parents (children often adapt more quickly than parents to a new environment and become sources of knowledge), employees, and citizens—leading to less participation or even withdrawal from school activities.

Given these factors, Deslandes argues that the attitudes and behaviour of school staff (e.g., implicit and explicit stereotyping or body language) have more of an impact on the school-family relationship than do language barriers. It is critical to remember that most immigrants come to Canada for a better life—for their children especially. They value education highly and want their children to succeed in this new country. However, immigrant parents sometimes feel that their own values and culture are rapidly being replaced as their children are quickly inundated and in constant contact with (sometimes) new values. Given all this information, the school has an important role to play!

Key findings from the study that can be applied to a healthy school community include the following:

- Person-to-person contact. Encourage face-to-face meetings as much as possible (use an interpreter if necessary) and involve parents in decision making to ensure that parents feel that their voice is valued and understood. Immigrant parents, their culture, and their communities deserve to be included and respected. Consider how this can happen in your school.
- Fear of offending authority figures. Immigrant parents often feel the need to communicate without creating conflict because there may have been serious repercussions for causing conflict in the past. This can mean that issues of racism, slander, or bullying can go unreported as parents try to downplay these incidents so they and their children do not stand out. Make clear to all parents and students that harassment or disrespectful treatment of others will not be tolerated.
- Intergenerational conflict. The more that culture and values differ between an immigrant's country of origin and those of mainstream Canada, the more likely there will be conflict between children and parents regarding dress, food, educational expectations, and opportunities for interaction. Be aware of when and how these conflicts may happen and be prepared to address them up front—but with diplomacy and cultural sensitivity.

- Community involvement. Immigrant parents tend to be very involved with their cultural community. Intercultural suppers, dances, and other performances can form a bridge between cultures and foster appreciation and understanding of cultural differences.
- Extra-curricular activities. Deslandes argues that the most consistent practice for family involvement in the school is through sport, excursions, performances, and even invitations to give in-class presentations about cultural practices. These activities are a prime opportunity to create intercultural understanding and respect. They also help immigrant parents feel that they are valued members of the school community.

A final point that Deslandes makes is that, "for teachers, it is important not to base one's conclusions only on parents' actions, but to look for the *meaning* behind the practice." It is easy to notice the practice or action, but it takes time, understanding, and relationship building to get a deeper sense of the underlying meaning and rationale. When a school community endeavours to create an environment where deeper understanding of cultural practices is encouraged, it is possible to "develop conditions that promote the development of effective partnerships between immigrant families and the school."

PHE Canada has an excellent resource that uses an asset-based community development approach to support immigrant children in becoming more physically active. We Belong offers tools and ideas to facilitators of after-school programs to increase participation of new Canadians in physical activities. —PHE Canada, Ottawa

Case Study

By Doug Gleddie

Inner-city schools in Canadian urban centres have some of the most diverse student populations in the world.

Schools in these areas can expect classes to reflect a rich diversity in terms of race, socioeconomic status, immigration or refugee status, gender, sexual orientation, religion, and dis/abilities.

In your role (which you may define as you wish) at a large urban K-9 school, you *think* that you *accept* students, *respect* them, and *recognize* their identities and needs in a genuine way. And you're trying to create a culturally relevant healthy school climate that engages *everyone* in health.

However, since students, parents, and school staff all come from diverse backgrounds, it can be difficult at times to promote the values of *acceptance, respect,* and *recognition.*

1 Beginning with the framework of the four Fs—friends, family, finances, and fitting in—how will you ensure that your healthy school is truly an inviting destination for everyone?

2 How would you incorporate and support a diversity of voices in authentic, respectful, and constructive ways? Consider the four pillars of the JCSH framework.

3 This chapter identifies several vulnerabilities for children in families of low socio-economic status. How can your healthy school help to "fill the gaps" in these areas? Be specific! If possible, use a concrete example from your context and apply some of the strategies featured in this chapter to help you get started while being mindful of privacy and confidentiality issues.

4 Consider how you might design a project or an event that uses health as a way to understand the diversity of cultures in your school.

It's Your Turn

1. Initiate a survey or questionnaire in your school community (or use existing data from the school district) to assess the variety of cultural backgrounds and practices. Present the results at a staff meeting and initiate a discussion about how to make best use of this information.
2. Use a shared format such as Google Drive to collaboratively create a database of health and social supports for school staff and parents and guardians to access. Share the database on your school website.

✓ Action Checklist

Individual	Suggested Follow-up
Pre-service Teacher	❑ Make an audio or video recording of a few of your lessons and assess them for affirmations and prohibitions. ❑ Research the social supports available for your practicum community and share your findings at a staff meeting. ❑ Take time to become familiar with the variety of cultures represented at your school and plan lessons accordingly.
Health and Physical Education Teacher	❑ Ensure that your lessons and activities are culturally relevant. ❑ When providing intramural or club-type activities, be aware of cultural and socioeconomic differences. Address these from a strengths-based perspective. ❑ Assess your program and instruction practices using the four Fs. Are you doing enough to be inclusive and show respect for diversity? ❑ Assess your program from an affirmations and prohibitions standpoint. How can you help develop strong, independent learners?
Administrator	❑ Become familiar with the social supports available at a variety of levels (school district, community, city, province/territory). ❑ Invite elders or cultural representatives to speak to school staff and students about healthy practices. ❑ Provide teachers with key information about affirmations and prohibitions and design a school-wide framework for increasing affirmations.
Parent / Guardian	❑ Consider your own culture, community, and background. What practices stand out as particularly healthy? If there are any unhealthy practices, how might these be minimized? ❑ Share and discuss your findings with your child and their teacher.
Health Promotion Coordinator (Health Sector)	❑ Provide a list of social support systems and organizations for school staff to refer to and access. ❑ Make clear and evidence-based connections between strong social supports and academic success.

Chapter 6 Summary

Schools represent a society's most promising opportunity to inspire citizens to make their communities a better place. A school is much more than bricks and mortar. It is the people of the school community who bring learning to life. A multitude of positive outcomes are possible when all members of that community—teachers, students, parents, guardians, business and community leaders, elders, and public health workers—assume a shared responsibility for education. Even more positive results can be achieved when the health of the school community is the school's cornerstone. Students benefit from the collective wisdom and experiences of others when all members of the school community are actively engaged in promoting health and wellness. Students feel supported not only at school, but when they are away from school as well. To be effective, healthy schools must be inviting and welcoming. This can often be a challenge when schools are under pressure to restrict public access for safety reasons. However, a healthy school will explore opportunities to overcome these barriers (some real and some perceived) in a way that continues to ensure student safety while also recognizing the vital importance of establishing social supports and partnerships with the wider community.

Questions for Reflection

1 Identify individuals or organizations in your community that could be key members of a healthy school committee. Be sure to consider all relevant stakeholders and the type of support they might provide.

2 What can families do in terms of actions and activities to help support and reinforce key health knowledge that students obtain within a healthy school?

3 Cultural traditions and customs can have both positive and negative influences on an individual's health. At what point might health concerns supersede cultural practices and beliefs? Provide an example from your own reading or experience.

4 Identify potential barriers—real or perceived—that often discourage members of the school community from becoming actively involved in health-promoting initiatives. How might these barriers be overcome to help ensure that social supports are in place to nurture a healthy school environment? How can members of the school community help develop and implement a plan to overcome such barriers?

5 What kinds of tools and resources might help busy, overworked parents or guardians feel more informed about and connected to their children's learning experiences?

6 What kinds of practices and strategies might help various members of a school community reduce high stress levels and cope better with the challenges of balancing school, work, and family obligations? How might these practices and strategies be shared amongst members of the school community?

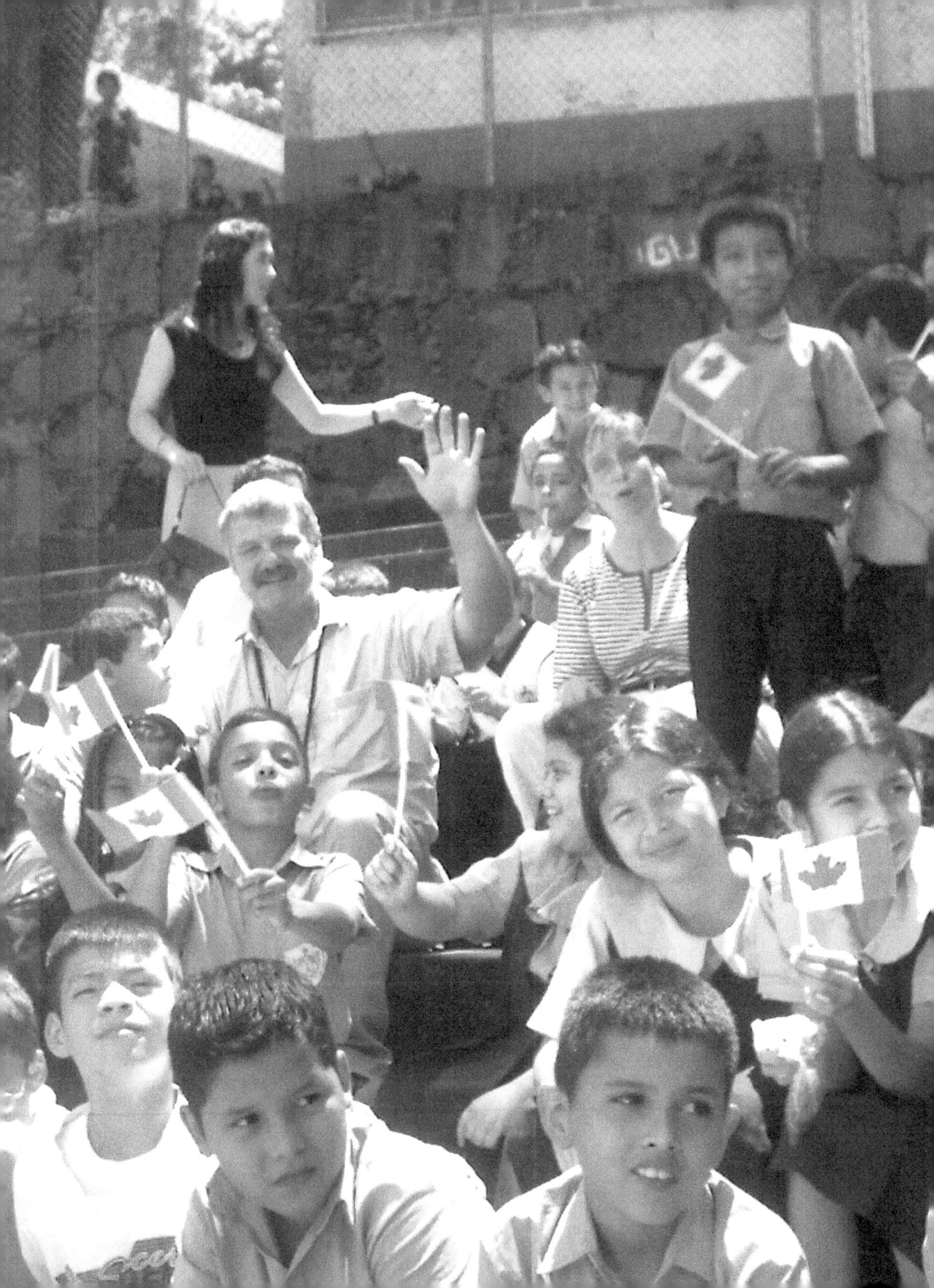

7

Looking to the Future

Building on the past

Much of the content in the previous chapters embodies Andy Anderson's original work that he managed to complete during the later stages of his illness. Andy's legacy and leadership in the area of health-promoting schools has endured to this day. This final chapter highlights various healthy school initiatives that have built on Andy's work and that have preserved and refined his vision and his legacy in many significant ways.

These "living examples" demonstrate that Andy's spirit lives on and inspires people in communities around the world. The profiles of health-promoting school initiatives were contributed by people and organizations who had the opportunity to work with and learn from Andy and who have made a commitment to ensure that his work and ideas continue to influence wise policies, best practices, and healthy relationships in schools each and every day.

Ever Active Schools: A Provincial Example (Alberta)

By Doug Gleddie, *Associate Professor, Faculty of Education, University of Alberta; Former Director, Ever Active Schools (2004–2010),*

Once upon a time, in the year 2000, there was a prairie province that decided to help kids become more active in schools. The province wanted to see a movement in schools that would create a healthy school community so kids could learn in environments that support physical activity. The province asked the Health and Physical Education Council (HPEC)—a very cool group of teachers from the Alberta Teachers' Association—to bring together some caring and knowledgeable people to complete this sentence: "If a school was a healthy, active school, there would be/ you would see...." The people consulted, who were from villages and cities across the province, responded to the group leader's question with wonderful ideas and suggestions. They wrote down their responses eagerly and knowledgably as they were teachers, parents, guardians, superintendents, health professionals, and consultants who had lots of good ideas. After reviewing all of their ideas, the leader from HPEC looked far and wide around the world for the perfect model to match all the people's good ideas. Lo and behold, they found that program in Active Australia. So the leader shouted, "Hooray! Today we have discovered a model for our own healthy, active school program. It shall be called Ever Active Schools (EAS)." And the people cheered. Over the next few years, EAS also moved from a focus on physical activity to embracing a Comprehensive School Health (CSH) philosophy and model.

EAS was an energetic and effective program. The people really liked the letter E (because that is what "Ever Active" began with). So they formed other "E" words that described how to become a healthy, active school. Originally these E words included Education, Everyone, Everywhere, and Environment, but because all good things grow and change, in 2007 they reassessed the 4 Es and adapted them to the current 4 Es, which are:

- Everyone. collaborating in a meaningful way with the people involved in the everyday life of the school and ensuring equal and inclusive opportunities for everyone to make healthy choices
- Education. supporting a culture of learning for all school community members, including wellness-related programs for students and health-promotion learning opportunities for teachers, staff, and parents and guardians
- Environment. fostering safe social and physical environments in the school, home, and community; implementing policies that enable healthy active lifestyles; and cultivating a place where everyone knows they belong
- Evidence. collaboratively identifying goals, planning for action, and gathering information to indicate the effectiveness of actions to support healthy active lifestyles throughout the school community

Now, when the leader began to implement the program across the land, people were afraid of the change that they thought would result. The teachers asked, "How can I do one more thing in my school? I am already doing too much!" They were also afraid to enter the gymnasium and find themselves amidst throngs of energized children trying new and wonderful activities. The principals asked: "How can I afford to do this?" The students, well, the students weren't asked... yet! Ever Active helped schools find the answers. They trained the teachers so they were no longer afraid. They explained to the principals that the concept of Comprehensive School Health (CSH) is not about money—it is about mindset. And they encouraged the schools to talk to their students so they could be involved in bringing about positive changes in their schools. EAS identified leaders across the land and shared promising practices with them to increase physical activity for Alberta students so they could help the principals and teachers solve many problems. The leader knew that having students learn in healthy, active schools would help students live happily ever active....

The children at EAS schools were, indeed, very active students. However, EAS knew that it is also important for healthy kids to eat well, play well, and get along with others. They began to support healthy eating and mental well-being initiatives as well. EAS showed school communities that health issues can be looked at through a CSH lens, and Ever Active was an example of a really effective CSH program. In fact, for EAS schools, CSH is just the way we do business!

Not just any school can become an Ever Active School. The school has to look clearly and critically at what it is currently doing by completing a thorough review. Parents, guardians, students, teachers, administrators, and other folks involved in the school all need to review the features of the school by using the assessment tool provided by EAS. All the people who review the school then create an Action Plan to make sure lots of good things begin to happen at the school. Then they tell the EAS leader how they are doing by reassessing themselves each year so schools can ask themselves if they have succeeded or not, and what criteria they are using to determine success or lack of success, so schools can ask themselves if they have succeeded or not.

Ever Active Schools was developed by school communities to meet the needs of all Alberta school communities. And the program was so well-liked that three government ministries have supported the implementation of Ever Active Schools in Alberta: Alberta Education, Alberta Health and Wellness, and Alberta Tourism, Parks and Recreation.

Now one of the premier CSH programs across the land, EAS has grown and expanded its horizons. Schools across Alberta have access to a wide variety of services and supports for physical activity, healthy eating, mental well-being, and student leadership in schools.

One of the most fun events planned by EAS are the Healthy Active School Symposia (HASS), designed to bring students, teachers, parents, guardians, administrators, and community stakeholders together as a team from each participating school to share promising practices, plan goals as a team, and mentor one another. This annual event has become so popular that regional sessions are now held across Alberta.

A giant in the land, Andy Anderson, was talking about Ever Active Schools one day and he said, "Ever Active Schools is the sweet spot on the CSH racquet." This was indeed high praise from the giant who was viewed as the leading expert in Canada on health-promoting schools and whose opinion was held in high esteem by educators around the world. Ever Active Schools has been growing ever since!

Inspired by Andy's leadership and vision for CSH in Canada and around the world, EAS founded an annual Healthy Schools conference entitled Shaping the Future. The conference has been held very successfully each year since that first January in 2010 and is recognized by all stakeholders as this country's premier healthy schools conference.

Healthy Schools: A Provincial Example (Ontario)

By the Ontario Health and Physical Education Association (Ophea)

Kids love nutritious foods. They like exercise, too. Don't believe it? Just talk to one of the students at a certified Ophea Healthy School. Stop by John McRae Public School in Markham, Ontario, for example. The excitement in the air is palpable each week as students prepare for their "Wednesday Walk"—a 25-minute outdoor excursion led by the principal, which winds its way through the neighbourhood streets. Or check in on the kids at J.R. Henderson School in Kingston, Ontario as they play in their new community-built schoolyard, complete with a garden, gazebo, volleyball courts, a mini-putt golf course, and a fitness trail. Ask the kids at Bishop Gallagher Senior Elementary School in Thunder Bay, Ontario, if they like "Fruity Fridays." Or see how the Grade 5 students at Gateway Public School in Toronto respond to playing sports with a bunch of police officers every Thursday afternoon.

These are all examples of Ophea-certified Healthy Schools, and they're a testament to the shift toward healthy living that can come about when educators, students, and community partners all work together to achieve common goals.

The Organization

Since 1921, Ophea has been working to support the health and learning of children and youth in Ontario. Ophea is a not-for-profit organization that champions healthy, active living in schools and communities through quality programs and services, partnerships, and advocacy, and it is guided by the vision that all children and youth deserve, value, and enjoy the lifelong benefits of healthy, active living. Operating up to 30 projects annually that are both provincial and national in scope, Ophea serves approximately 2.1 million children and youth in Ontario.

The Challenge

Ophea recognizes that Ontario's children are at risk of being the first generation to have a lower life expectancy than their parents. Some risks leading to chronic diseases are modifiable, such as tobacco use, harmful use of alcohol, unhealthy diet, and physical inactivity. The challenge for Ophea was threefold: How can we encourage our kids to eat a healthy diet, increase their physical activity, and avoid smoking in a way that will empower them to take personal responsibility for those actions not just now, but throughout their lives?

This is where Ophea's Healthy Schools Certification comes in. An Ophea-certified Healthy School involves the entire school community coming together to share ideas, set goals, and take action. In fact, when the entire school community takes responsibility for its choices, the changes become an intrinsic part of the fabric of the school's culture. It's an approach that involves all community members and partners—and at its very heart are the students.

The Healthy Schools mindset involves empowering students so their voices can be heard. By engaging students in leadership opportunities, they'll come to realize at an early age that their choices and actions can have a deep impact on themselves, their peers, their classrooms, their school, and their community. When we can come together and establish this leadership incentive, young people are better equipped to meet the challenges of today. They will also be empowered to make healthier choices and to manage the risks they will face, whatever they may be, well into the future.

The secret to healthier kids does not exist in a standard program; rather, it requires helping kids take control of their own well-being—and that, in essence, is the Healthy Schools approach.

The Approach

Ophea's Healthy Schools Certification engages entire school communities—students, parents, guardians, school staff, public health agencies, and the school board—in promoting and enhancing the health and well-being of children, youth, and the broader community.

By means of a comprehensive and consultative process, Healthy Schools plan and implement activities and strategies to address the specific health-related topics identified by the school community. Since every community has different needs, the secret to enabling kids to be healthier does not exist in establishing a one-size-fits-all program. The Healthy Schools approach empowers schools to implement activities and strategies that will make their communities healthier, based on decisions made by the very children and youth involved.

Instead of imposing rules and policies to push kids to become healthier, the Healthy Schools approach teaches students to work with their teachers, parents, guardians, and the community to become empowered to make healthy choices for themselves. Whether they're in the schoolyard, the classroom, or the lunchroom, students emerge as the leaders and the decision makers.

While the primary audience is made up of teachers and educators, it is Ophea's unique student engagement strategy that contributes to the overall success of the Healthy Schools approach.

The Problem

There is no shortage of individuals and organizations that want to help solve Canada's health and physical activity shortfall. Schools all over the country are attempting to become "healthy," but there is no one-size-fits-all program that is going to prove successful across different school communities. A valid approach in Northern Ontario might fail miserably in Eastern Ontario or in a different province altogether.

Further complicating matters is the fact that school communities don't always have the necessary resources to engage students in both identifying the challenges and the actions required to support healthy, active living within their school and beyond.

The Solution

Over the past 20 years, Ophea has led the successful implementation of multiple school-based health research projects that show that the Healthy Schools approach works. Based on the results of these third-party academic studies conducted in relation to healthy school initiatives, schools adopting this approach in Ontario saw the following changes:

- increased physical activity levels and trends toward healthier eating behaviours among both students and teachers (Living School)
- positive change in the school health environment relating to tobacco control, physical activity, and healthy eating (Lungs Are For Life)
- schools that had higher school health environment scores in physical activity were more likely to have students who were physically active for 90 minutes or more each day (Lungs Are For Life)
- lower likelihood of students' use of tobacco products (Smoke-Free Ontario, Year 1 Preliminary Findings)
- higher exposure to anti-tobacco messages and higher participation in anti-smoking activities (Smoke-Free Ontario, Year 1 Preliminary Findings)

While many tools are available to help Ontario's schools adopt a healthy schools approach, schools still face the challenge of doing so in a planned and purposeful way. To address these challenges, Ophea developed Healthy Schools Certification, which provides schools with a process that puts the healthy schools approach into action and publicly recognizes the school's achievements.

Ophea's Healthy Schools Certification is based on the Healthy Schools approach that is recognized by the World Health Organization and it aligns with the Ontario Ministry of Education's Foundations for a Healthy School resource. Ophea employed a thorough process to develop Ontario's Healthy Schools Certification, including a research/needs assessment, a concept test, and an external review.

The Ontario Healthy Schools Certification process consists of the following 6 steps:

- Step 1. Identify your school team (existing or new)
- Step 2. Assess school assets, needs, and opportunities
- Step 3. Identify your priority health topic (e.g., healthy eating, physical activity, tobacco avoidance, sufficient sleep and rest, substance use)
- Step 4. Develop an action plan
- Step 5. Take action and monitor progress
- Step 6. Celebrate and reflect

Schools earn points at each step in the process and are recognized for their achievements through a Gold, Silver, or Bronze Certification (www.ophea.net/hscertification). By completing the 6-Step Healthy Schools Process over the course of the school year, registered schools will earn points and can apply to be certified in April as a Gold-, Silver-, or Bronze-level Healthy School.

Certification is based on a school's ability to follow and complete the process, and not on the type or number of activities chosen. This process guides a school community through the planning and implementation of a range of activities designed to reflect a selected priority health topic. The process is annual, repeated each school year, and it is sufficiently flexible for all communities across Ontario to sustain it year over year.

Simply put, the Healthy Schools approach empowers school communities to follow a simple, step-by-step process to change their school for the better. Individual schools that follow this process report on their progress and are then formally certified as a Healthy School and recognized for their work.

Every school in Ontario has the potential to become a Healthy School. All they need are the tools and support to get there. Our mandate is to provide supports to build their capacity to implement this process on an annual basis.

As the Healthy Schools approach grows to encompass all 5,000 Ontario schools, Ophea will collaborate with school boards, schools, parents, guardians, public health units, and community partners to facilitate this approach. Our work focuses on supporting school leaders to understand and apply our tools so that they, in turn, can empower their students to take action on the issues that are most important to them.

The Social Impact of Healthy Schools

The benefits of undertaking the process to become a Healthy School make it worthwhile. There are numerous examples across Ontario of schools and communities working together in this way and seeing tremendous results.

These results include increased physical activity and trends toward healthier eating (for both students and teachers); increased student attentiveness, alertness, and attendance; higher test scores, a reduction in behavioural issues; and a stronger sense of student belonging, attachment, and safety within the school community.

APPLE Schools—Comprehensive School Health Works (A Provincial Example)

By Marg Schwartz, *APPLE Schools, Alberta*

The Alberta Project Promotion active Living and healthy Eating in Schools (APPLE Schools) began in 2007 as a philanthropically funded initiative operating under the direction of Dr. Paul Veugelers, Professor and Canada Research Chair at the University of Alberta, School of Public Health. The project was piloted in ten vulnerable schools in the Edmonton region, with one school located in Athabasca, Alberta. The project design incorporated the implementation of a Comprehensive School Health (CSH) approach to creating a healthy school community, designed to impact the home, school, and community in positive ways, as this approach is recognized internationally as being the most effective process for addressing health behaviours in a school setting (Veugelers and Schwartz, 2010).

Only 30% of Grade 5 kids in Alberta eat enough fruits and vegetables (Veugelers: 2014). Obesity rates have reached 8.1%, an increase from the 7.3% observed in 2012. The prevalence of overweight (excluding obese) students reached 21.3%. Only 9% of Canadian kids get enough physical activity (ParticipACTION, 2015). Obesity has tripled and chronic diseases are being reported at younger and younger ages (Veugelers and Schwartz, 2010). Based on these statistics, we need to look at the issue of adult chronic diseases as a pediatric concern and start developing healthy habits at a young age—which is the premise underlying APPLE Schools.

In 2007, the existing provincial organization providing support and leadership was Ever Active Schools. Therefore, APPLE Schools utilized the terminology and resources of Ever Active Schools to help school staff, parents, guardians, students, and community partners develop a healthy school community.

The project incorporated design elements that characterized the successful Annapolis Valley Health Promoting School Project (AVHPSP) in Nova Scotia (Veugelers and Fitzgerald, 2005), which had expanded from its original seven schools to all 40 schools in the Annapolis Valley Regional School Board. Participants' experience with the AVHPSP indicated the importance of a continuous presence in the schools and, therefore, the APPLE Schools project tailored intervention strategies to each of its schools. Since the APPLE Schools project was well-funded, the intervention pilot included full-time School Health Facilitators placed in each of the schools to address the unique needs and barriers associated with healthy eating and physical activity. APPLE Schools was the first school health-promotion research project to include full-time School Health Facilitators in each school for an extended time frame: three-and-a-half years, with a decrease to a 0.2 Full Time Equivalent (FTE) in year four.

The project's goals were to increase physical activity and healthy eating in school-aged children, to increase the capacity of the school community to address health-related behaviours, and to foster healthy school environments. These strategies would ultimately feed into the longer-term goals to prevent overweight and reduce the risk of chronic disease (Schwartz, 2010).

In November 2007, ten School Health Facilitators (SHF) were hired and trained for six weeks prior to the program's implementation in selected schools in January 2008. Because there was no syllabus available for training staff to implement Comprehensive School Health, an entire curriculum was developed. (Storey, Montemerro, and Schwartz., 2015). The goals of training went beyond the basics of learning successful health-promotion strategies and tapping into local supports and services. An additional goal of developing a strong team bond was paramount for the success of the project, as health promotion in schools is not for the faint of heart.

The importance of a strong team of SHFs became apparent as the team members moved into the individual schools and were immediately struck with how their role was isolated in relation to any other role in the school. The SHFs were graduates from programs of education, physical education, nutritional sciences (RD), psychology, and marketing. When asked what degree would best prepare students for becoming a SHF, I replied that a degree in "relationship building" is the most important element for success. The most imperative need was to work with an entire school community as well as to work together and support one another as SHFs.

APPLE Schools change the paradigm of schools and school cultures so that health becomes a priority and an integral part of everyday business. Health is taught, is visible, and is present in all aspects of the school environment—from the foods that are served and sold, to the ways in which students treat each other and include everyone as part of the school community. The core concept is to reach all kids, not just those who like to move or who are already eating well and feeling included. The entire school community becomes engaged in being aware of healthful habits and role modelling of healthy living behaviours. In a healthy school, health is taken into account when planning celebrations, rewards, and parental events. It essentially becomes part of the fabric of what the school stands for and does each and every day.

How is a healthy school culture achieved? It starts with a conversation. Because school staff will often tell you there is no time for conversations as they are so busy in their classrooms, the role of the SHF is key to starting the conversations. Conversations are sparked at staff meetings, at meetings with parents and guardians, in the classrooms, during the organization of student leadership teams, and during assemblies. There are conversations with the school nurse and local recreation practitioners, the parent who teaches yoga, and the grandmother or grandfather who runs the snack program. The conversations are key to taking the crucial first steps.

So why isn't every school a healthy school? If asked, virtually all schools would say they care a great deal about health, but our experience in APPLE Schools has shown that unless schools are provided with support to overcome the barriers of time, money, and knowledge, schools find it difficult to prioritize health as a result of so many competing priorities that demand attention. A healthy school is not "done to you" but is created by all. Schools should not be afraid to take on the challenge of creating healthy environments as parents and students tend to strongly support healthy school policy. In fact, over 90% of parents have indicated support of both healthy nutrition and physical activity policies (Spitters, 2009).

The Results of the Pilot Project

After two years of intervention at the pilot schools, the Grade 5 students measured in each school had increased their vegetable and fruit intake by 10%. Obesity was reduced by 14%. Physical activity increased to reach provincial averages after starting well below those averages. (Fung, 2012). Further research has demonstrated that the programming occurring in APPLE Schools increased physical activity by 35%, particularly in inactive populations, which in turn addresses health inequities in the schools. (Vander Ploeg, Maximova, McGavock, and Veugelers, 2014). For copies of the evaluation tools used in APPLE Schools, see www.realkidsalberta.ca.

Process evaluation conducted by Dr. Kate Storey of the School of Public Health also defined the importance of leadership and the role of the school administrator in the implementation of CSH (Roberts, 2015). This research helped to engage the school administrators in the project and demonstrated the significance of role models and leaders who will champion all initiatives occurring in the schools.

There is a strong focus on student leadership within APPLE Schools and a preliminary study demonstrated a clear linkage between well-developed leadership skills and health habits (Ferland, 2015), which helped schools understand the importance of involving children's voices and leadership in developing well-accepted implementation strategies.

The research also has indicated a positive return on investment, something that is rarely calculated in health-promotion strategies. Preliminary estimates reported by Dr. Veugelers at the National Forum on Public Health, University of Alberta, in November 2013 stated that for every dollar spent in APPLE Schools, the government saves $13 in avoided future health-care costs associated with obesity. Dr. Veugelers also published data indicating that if APPLE Schools were up-scaled across Alberta, between $33 and $82 million could be saved annually in avoided health-care costs (Tran, 2014).

There was noted improvement in academic achievement seen in an internal review, particularly in provincial achievement in mathematics and language arts. (Nadirova, 2014)

The uniqueness of the research undertaken within the project does not end with the scientific publications. After each year of data collection, the school received a school report outlining the results of the research conducted on their Grade 5 students, parents and guardians, and administrators. A sampling of health behaviours (e.g., vegetable and fruit consumption, sleep habits, and family eating habits) compared to other APPLE Schools as well as 150 randomly selected schools was reported in an easy-to-read format and sent to each school administrator. Sessions were then held with school administrators that focused on how they could use the real-time data to educate parents, guardians, and staff on specific gains or identified issues. For example, one administrator was astounded to find out that 47% of her parents reported that they were concerned that money would not be available to buy food in their household. This finding prompted the administrator to immediately stop charging parents for field trips and other whole-school events. The use of evidence to improve practice is a guiding principle for the project.

Immediate changes to each school's action plans based on the research results allowed the focus of the project to continue to evolve within each school community. A clear example of this was the initial positive result of improving physical activity levels. The data indicated that the greatest increase in physical activity was occurring in the most active populations. The focus for the ensuing year therefore became a reorganization of all physical activity events to be designed to reach the students who were previously not engaged. Once schools began to identify the disengaged students, these students were asked to provide input into which activities would interest them. The resulting increases in physical activity were strongly demonstrated not only in school, but in after-school hours and on weekends (Vander Ploeg, Wu, McGavock, and Veugelers, 2014).

Activities chosen to improve mental well-being, physical activity, and healthy eating are at the discretion of each school, as they created an action plan with input from all stakeholders, including parents, guardians, students, staff, and community members. (For specific examples, ideas, resources, and videos of strategies used in APPLE Schools, see www.appleschools.ca.)

By 2014, the project had expanded to over 50 schools in northern Alberta and a separate foundation was established to obtain funding from a variety of corporate and philanthropic interests.

Lessons Learned

- Lesson 1. There were many lessons learned since 2007, the first one being that health promotion in schools is hard, slow work. The skill set of the School Health Facilitator is directly correlated to how difficult it is to move the culture and the speed at which this can be accomplished (Storey, Spitters, et al., 2011). As a result, maintaining the morale of the SHF team is essential to help them navigate difficult issues. As one example, early in an intervention, excited students arrived at a SHF's office door to invite the facilitator to a "chicken party" that was taking place in their classroom. The SHF thought that the teacher had finally taken out the rubber chicken activity box provided to the class The sense of disappointment was extreme when the facilitator walked into the classroom to find that the teacher had organized a fried chicken and pop party! However, this incident led to a frank discussion with the school administrator, who felt that it was time to start developing health policy to ensure that all teachers were engaged in the concept of striving to become a healthy school. So, the first lesson is to ensure that health-promotion practitioners are supported by a culture conducive to understanding that health promotion is not a steady upward climb, but more like meandering along a river filled with twists and turns. A rock in the middle of the river is not viewed as impeding progress, but as an opportunity to re-route the search to find smoother channels to explore.
- Lesson 2. People want to be heard. Most health promotion in schools begins with discussions. Some of the discussions are difficult: for example, finding ways to gain teachers' trust and understanding so they will re-think providing candy as a reward or helping them understand that cancelling physical education is not conducive to positive health and learning outcomes. Opportunities for

discussions with staff and parents and guardians must be both purposeful and skillfully designed so that even the quiet voices can be heard and can become a vital part of the conversation. The project only becomes ubiquitous when everyone feels they are part of the solution.

- Lesson 3. Evidence is powerful. When a school received a school report indicating that over 57% of their students were using electronics in their bedrooms after the parents expected them to be asleep, staff and parents reacted quickly to try to address this health concern. The parents and staff became motivated to implement a "Be A Sleep Star" campaign using bulletin boards, morning announcements, newsletters to parents on ways to improve sleep habits, and classroom activities for teachers to teach the related concepts. The resulting strategies were implemented and then measured the following year. Seeing changes as a result of the strategies they had designed was most rewarding and meaningful. The research also helped with individual school issues. For example, one school was resistant to engaging all staff to increase the quality and quantity of learning opportunities related to health. Their school report showed that when parents and students were surveyed on their health knowledge (e.g., how many minutes of physical activity should be achieved each day or how many fruits and vegetables should be eaten), the results indicated that parents scored higher than the students. The administrator then provided stronger leadership and professional development was received by all teachers to improve quality learning experiences based on health-related curricula. Evidence is key to providing motivation for change.
- Lesson 4. Health is personal. The very presence of a health-promotion staff person in a school makes people think about their own health habits. Occasionally, some people become defensive or feel that they are being told they "can't" do something (which is never the APPLE Schools message). It is important to respect the opinions of others and to slowly engage them over a period of time. We experienced many examples of chopping fresh peppers for a taste-testing event, and overheard comments that it is a shame to go to all that work when the teachers felt sure the students wouldn't eat them. In fact, the students not only ate all of the peppers, but they licked the hummus bowl clean! Therefore, our advice is to meet people where they are and to start from whatever level of awareness they may possess.
- Lesson 5. Don't reinvent the wheel. There are many, many partners in CSH. Use of existing policies, resources, tools, and support provided by others makes good sense. Wasting time in creating a new physical activity when there are literally thousands of resources available is not practical. If school staff and parents and guardians are directed to the myriad of resources available and when the project moves to a level of maintenance and sustainability, the resources are still accessible. We use Canadian-focused resources, particularly in terms of nutrition education materials. The use of "approved" materials is very important in maintaining a consistent message. CSH is complicated, so

consistent terminology and focusing is key; for example, teaching students and parents the terminology used for nutrition guidelines for their province makes it easier to keep everyone "on the same page" when devising nutrition messages.

- Lesson 6. Ask yourself "Who is not there"? This concept is one of the key guiding principles required for success. Making the fit students fitter is not the goal of a well-planned health-promotion strategy! If a nutrition campaign is being run to encourage students to include fresh vegetables in their lunches, for example, then ensure that you have fresh vegetables available for all students to access so that those students who are unable to receive fresh vegetables at home can still "play the game" and be part of the process.
- Lesson 7. Ask, "What can you do?" Health promotion in schools is not about moving mountains in a hurry. It takes many small steps by many people before the movement becomes significant. Celebrating every small step is important. Congratulate those teachers who make the change from candy rewards to non-food rewards. Instead of focusing on those who are not engaged, work with those who are supportive and a critical mass will be reached over time. It is important, however, to help everyone understand that changing the culture of a school is not the "job" of the SHF. There is a role for every student, parent/guardian, staff member, and community member to make small changes. Change occurs slowly and it will probably take at least two years of health-promotion strategies before there is a readiness to develop a wellness policy to address health within an entire school community. Be patient. Change will happen.
- Lesson 8. Nothing moves without administrators' support. The role of leadership in the school is essential to changing a school's culture. There is also a documented process that administrators seem to follow before they become role-modelling champions (Roberts, 2015). Two meetings each year are scheduled with administrators to set goals for the year and to review the annual results. As well, two meetings are hosted annually for all administrators to gather for professional learning related to their role as administrator in an APPLE Schools program and to engage administrators in a network of professionals who are all working toward similar goals. Because administrators tend to move to new schools every three to four years, it is important to engage and educate school leaders continuously to ensure sustainability.

After eight years, it is exciting to see the sustainable changes evident in all 50 schools. Every APPLE School has developed and implemented a wellness-related policy. Every policy has been developed by the individual school community to meet the needs of that community. Each policy is different and unique. Policy as a product is far less important than the process used to develop the policy, as there are many discussions, revisions, and buy-in achieved throughout the process. Action plans, policies, and other guidelines produced by the schools are varied and ever-changing, which is consistent with a health-promotion cycle of assessment, implementation, evaluation, and renewal (Schwartz, 2010).

APPLE Schools is a unique and successful CSH project listed on the Public Health Agency of Canada's Best Practice portal. The National Cancer Institute has also posted APPLE Schools as a successful Research Tested Intervention Program. Both of these prestigious postings attest to the strong evidence base and the efficacy of health-promotion strategies employed in APPLE Schools. Dr. Andy Anderson would be proud to know that Canada has spearheaded this internationally recognized and immensely successful project.

Healthy School Communities (A National Example)

By Physical and Health Education Canada (PHE Canada)

Physical and Health Education Canada (PHE Canada) is Canada's premier national professional organization for physical and health educators. Established in 1933, PHE Canada works closely with provincial and territorial health and physical education associations and partner organizations to deliver policy standards, develop resources and curriculum support tools, and advocate for issues that influence the healthy development of children and youth.

PHE Canada's Vision

"...All children and youth in Canada living healthy, physically active lives."

PHE Canada strives to achieve its vision by encouraging schools and school jurisdictions to become more comprehensive in their approach to school health. By advocating for and supporting the advancement of quality Health and Physical Education programs, we believe students will be equipped to develop the knowledge, skills, and attitudes needed to lead physically active and healthy lives, now and in their future.

In 2008, PHE Canada renamed its young professional award the Dr. Andy Anderson Young Professional Award in recognition of Andy's vast contributions to the healthy schools movement. Each year, PHE Canada awards this prestigious honour to one early-career professional in each province who best epitomizes exemplary work on behalf of the Physical and Health Education profession.

Healthy School Communities Initiative

A healthy school community increases student well-being and learning by promoting a culture of wellness for all members of the community. School administrators, educators, community partners, students, and parents and guardians all have a role to play in creating the healthy environment children require to be successful learners and empowered citizens.

PHE Canada's Healthy School Communities initiative is aimed at supporting school community efforts to ensure that all children and youth in Canada lead healthy, physically active lives. Through positive change in practices within the school community, children and youth will be nurtured to achieve their best—both in terms of academic progress and in their physical, emotional, and social development. A whole-school approach recognizes the relationship between health and learning, and when students are healthy, learning outcomes are positively affected.

Our current efforts are focused on:

- building awareness of the benefits of building healthy school communities and the existing frameworks that can support school efforts
- supporting local schools across Canada to become healthier by developing and implementing Healthy School Community plans, along with specific health-related projects, to move their schools toward healthier outcomes

- establishing Communities of Practice (COP) to share ideas, allow for collaboration, and provide mutual support for creating healthy school environments
- a Healthy School Communities National Forum designed to bring together community volunteers and professionals from the health, education, active living, and research sectors to connect with, celebrate, and learn from school communities who are working collaboratively to make healthy schools a priority

Antigua Champions for Health-Promoting Schools (An International Example)

By Dr. Joanna Sheppard, *Associate Professor, Faculty of Health Sciences, University of the Fraser Valley*

As part of the daily routine of the Champions for Health Promoting Schools program, a packed van of eager undergraduates from the Kinesiology and Physical Education department at the University of the Fraser Valley in Abbotsford, British Columbia prepare for their teaching day. Revising lesson plans, practising their open-ended questioning style, or just singing along to the Antiguan radio station, we motor along to one of nine Antigua, West Indies elementary schools with whom we have partnered for over eight years. Pulling up to the school, we are greeted by hundreds of excited children shouting, "The Canadians are here!" My undergraduate students are welcomed by tiny hands sliding into theirs as they share with their "new" Canadian teachers everything that has happened over the past year since they have been away and begin showing them around their school. I barely have a chance to tell my students what time I will be back to pick them up before they are fully involved in skipping, playing hand games, or swinging a cricket bat with the children.

However, in all of the commotion, one tug at my shirt about five years ago is a favourite program moment of mine. It was from a boy in Grade 3 who desperately wanted to tell me something. "Doctor Jo, do you remember last year when I used to be fat?" Stunned by the question, I began to stumble through a response only to be stopped mid-sentence by his next statement. Patting his belly, he said, "Well, you taught me last year how important it is to eat healthy and be active, and look at me now!" The little boy ran off to play and left me frozen for a moment. This moment made me realize the impact that the Champions for Health Promoting Schools program was having not only on the students in Antigua, but on everyone involved. This impact began with Dr. Andy Anderson.

The Champions Past

The Champions for Health Promoting Schools program was created 20 years ago by Dr. Andy Anderson. The reason for creating such a program is best explained through Andy's own words:

> School programs can play a vital role in the provision of learning opportunities that protect and promote the dignity of human life and freedom. Education can prepare young people to play active roles in their communities by empowering them to lead and responsibly manage change. Educational programs which enhance efforts to prepare young change agents with care for self and others in mind represent the forefront of educational improvement. (Anderson, 2006)

It was this passionate explanation that attracted members of the Ministry of Education in Antigua and Barbuda, the British Virgin Islands, and St. Vincent and the Grenadines. With the invitation and permission of the government of each of these countries and with the financial support of Scotiabank Canada, Andy and a team of his graduate students, including myself, Dr. James Mandigo, and Dr. Erin Hobin flew to each of these Caribbean Islands to lay the foundation of what is now known as the Champions for Health Promoting Schools Program (CHPS).

At that time, the CHPS program was dedicated to improving the life chances of children and their families throughout these three Caribbean countries by means of health and physical education initiatives. The program curriculum connected academic learning to caring for self, others, and the environment (Anderson, 2006). The Caribbean students learned about teamwork, self-esteem, positivity, self-care, and the environment, while at the same time learning various physical education skills such as net ball, rounders, skipping, games of tag, and so on. The program also paved the way to expand opportunities for Caribbean students to play leadership roles at school and in their communities, and to link community health projects with school projects.

For the first three years of the CHPS program, a small group of teacher candidates from the Ontario Institute for Studies in Education (O.I.S.E.) at the University of Toronto would embark to these three islands for six weeks in the spring to not only teach important health-promoting concepts surrounding the program, but also to practise their newly attained knowledge of classroom management and professional responsibility as a teacher on an international scale. As the CHPS program's momentum grew in positive ways, the untimely illness and death of our team leader Dr. Andy Anderson ground us to a halt as we mourned his passing. However, as promised, and with a new passion, dedication, and focus, the Champions for Health Promoting Schools Program launched a new chapter at the University of the Fraser Valley in British Columbia.

The Champions Present

For the past seven years, the Champions for Health Promoting Schools Program has been a collaborative effort between myself, a professor at the University of the Fraser Valley Kinesiology and Physical Education department in Abbotsford, British Columbia, and the Antigua/Barbuda Ministry of Education. With sustainable support from the Physical Education and Health and Family Life departments within the Antiguan Ministry, undergraduate students from the University of the Fraser Valley (also known as Champions) volunteer within nine elementary schools for a four-week placement. The Champions volunteer within the same elementary schools each year and are placed at one school for their full four-week program to gain the trust of their students and confidence in their teaching environments.

The foundation of this program is to teach the students of Antigua the life skills that can help them navigate through life's many challenges. The life skills as learned by the students and defined by the United Nations include communication and interpersonal skills; decision-making and critical thinking skills; and coping and self-management skills (UNICEF, 2012). Through months of preparation and the supportive guidance of Antiguan principals, the yearly Champions team consisting of between 22 to 26 undergraduate students creates, modifies, and perfects over 200 Health and Physical Education lesson plans reinforcing these life skills. More specifically, life skills embedded within the program focus on conflict resolution, patience, personal and social responsibility, sportspersonship, making healthy decisions, and taking ownership of one's environment. By means of game play and classroom work, Antiguan students are dynamically guided through individual, partner, and group activities toward an understanding of how and when a specific life skill may be needed. The Champions facilitate this understanding through the use of open-ended questions we call CCR.

Check-Connect-Reflect

As a way to determine whether the life skills teaching was fully understood by our Antiguan students, upon completion of the activity (whether physical or classroom-based), the Antiguan students are asked open-ended questions based upon what they have just learned. They are also asked how the lessons from the physical and health-related activities can be linked to their everyday lives. Our program calls this the CCR of the lesson—and it is the most important part of the lesson. The CCR open-ended questions not only assess understanding of the activity itself, but also assess how specific life skills can be applied in students' school and home environments.

An example of open-ended questions include:

Check:

- What skills did we work on in today's lesson?
- How did you communicate with your teammates within this game?

Connect:

- How do you communicate with your teacher and peers within the classroom?
- Why is it important to communicate with your teacher and peers?

Reflect:

- How do you communicate with your family members at home?
- In what ways can we communicate with our family members and our community?

By giving our Antiguan students an opportunity to voice their ideas and opinions, as stated over the numerous years by teachers and Antiguan colleagues alike, we allow our students to take ownership not only for their own actions but also for their words in all of the environments they inhabit.

Unity Games

Another important element of the CHPS program is the Unity Games Event. This event is best described as a Canadian sports day with a twist. The entire team of Champions is sent to one elementary school in the morning and to another school in the afternoon to play with the whole school population. Antiguan students participate in six physical activities, each of which highlights a different life skill (Sheppard & Wray, 2012). After each activity, Antiguan students discuss their actions using CCR through open-ended questions created by the Champions before they move on to the next activity. Not only is this a fun-filled day for both the Antiguan students and the Champions, but it is also an effective way for Antiguan teachers to participate and learn best practices that pertain to both physical-education and health-education environments.

Collaboration Is Key

Throughout the past 10 years, many positive connections and collaborations have been established and maintained within Antigua as well as in Canada. THE CHPS Champions have been invited annually to participate at the Antigua Barbuda Teacher's Union Professional Development Day, thereby enjoying an opportunity to collaborate with physical education and generalist teachers on the island through professional workshops presented by myself as well as by Antiguan educational specialists. We have volunteered with the Antiguan Wings Sports Club in both annual track and field meets and basketball tournaments. We have participated in many physical activity events across the islands, supporting and emphasizing the importance of living a healthy active life every day. The CHPS program has also financially supported the bi-yearly professional exchange visit of five Antiguan educators. For two weeks, our Antiguan colleagues attend lectures within the Kinesiology and Physical Education Department, are involved in practical teaching experiences with local physical and health educators as well as principals in British Columbia school boards, guest lecturing for our Champions for Health Promoting Schools program preparatory meetings, participating in a "Best Practices" workshop, as well as meeting key executives, faculty, and staff at the university. As a result of this collaboration, our Antiguan colleagues not only gain new knowledge from British Columbian educators that they then bring back to their country's classrooms, but they also share their own unique knowledge and experience from Antigua with the British Columbian educators.

Conclusion

Since the program's conception, over 150 undergraduate and graduate students from Canadian universities have been interacting positively with more than 5,000 Antiguan elementary students. However, I believe Antigua, including its students, teachers, and great friends, have truly impacted our Champions the most. In the words of a past Champion: "This program has truly been life-altering and I have learned so much about myself and about who I am as an educator. These life experiences will forever stay with me and I am so thankful that I am able to be a part of the Antigua Champions team."

With every new Champions team that is formed, Andy's legacy for Health Promoting Schools lives on both nationally and internationally. I encounter his passion, determination, and dedication within the students with whom I have collaborated in this program as well as within myself. Keeping Andy's legacy alive is attainable … as long as we remember that "Every Child Is a Champion!"

Final Thoughts

By James Mandigo

This concluding chapter represents what is possible when the healthy development of students and the school community are at the core of what a school does. The concepts associated with Health-Promoting Schools are relevant in communities across Canada and around the world. The examples provided in this chapter highlight the tremendous impact that Health-Promoting Schools continue to have in our communities, in our provinces and territories, in our country, and in our world. While the field of Health-Promoting Schools in Canada lost one of its greatest Champions when Dr. Andy Anderson passed away in 2007, the legacy of his work and ideas lives on in schools around the world. And that is really the goal of a Health Promoting School. When health is at the core foundation of any school, or any community for that matter, the benefits will continue to outlive us all.

I'm reminded of a story that a colleague of mine and a contributor to this book, Dr. John Corlett, once told to a group of pre-service teachers who had travelled to El Salvador to work with local teachers in finding ways to prevent youth violence. When he was young, John helped to plant a tree in his back yard. At the time, the tree was just a small sapling and barely noticeable. However, with care and nurturing, the tree grew bigger and stronger every year. When John returned to his childhood home forty years later, the tree had grown into a prominent feature of the back yard and had become a place to provide shade, host family gatherings, and provide hours of entertainment and recreational activities such as swinging and climbing. It had developed strong roots that had been able to withstand long, cold winters and fierce storms. The point of his story was that even though you may never get to see the full results of your work, investing your time and expertise to help make the world a healthier place is time well spent and it will pay social and spiritual dividends for years to come. This is why investing our time and energy in helping to make our school communities the healthiest they can be is not only beneficial in the present, but well into the future, too.

While brain cancer took a friend, colleague, husband, father, mentor, and teacher from us far too soon, the time that Andy devoted to advancing Health-Promoting Schools was time well spent and his efforts live on in school communities literally all around the world. If there is one idea that Andy would want us all to remember, I believe it would have been this: Investing our time, energy, and expertise in the health of our school communities can be one of the most rewarding gifts that we can give to others. We thank Andy for giving us this gift and we encourage all of you who have read this book to do the same. It is never wrong to do the right thing and the roots that you establish will continue to keep the tree of learning tall and strong for many years to come.

Epilogue

Thank you for reading this book. It has taken over four years to finally get this manuscript to a place where I am now proud of what I have to say. On a personal note, it is also especially important to me to have completed it, because six months ago I was diagnosed with a brain tumour that was later diagnosed as malignant. My first response when I thought of the book was, "I wish I could have finished it, but...." I am now at a point in my treatments where I see that the book has actually been written, will be published, and will find its way into your hands. I hope you will join me in celebrating the ideas and hopes that it represents in your classrooms, schools, and personal lives.

Andy Anderson
2007

Bibliography

Active Healthy Kids Canada (2013). Are we driving our kids to unhealthy habits? *The 2013 Active Healthy Kids Canada Report Card on Physical Activity for Children and Youth*. Toronto, ON. Available from: https://www.participaction.com/sites/default/files/downloads/Participaction-2013FullReportCard-UnhealthyHabits_1.pdf

Adamson, P. (2016). *Innocenti Report Card 11*. Florence: Unicef Office of Research.

Allensworth, D., Lawson, E., Nicholson, L., & Wyche, J. (1997). *Schools and health: Our nation's investment*. Washington, DC: National Academy.

Anderson, A. (2005). Understanding school improvement and school effectiveness from a health promoting school perspective. REICE. Revista Iberoamericana sobre Calidad, Eficacia y Cambio en Educación, 282–296.

Anderson, A. (2006). Health promoting schools: A community effort. *Physical and Health Education Journal*, 70(1).

Anderson, A., & Ronson, B. (2005). Democracy—the first principle of health promoting schools. *Journal of Health Education, 8,* 24–35.

Anderson, A., & Ronson, B. (2010). Democracy: The first principle of health promoting schools. In J. M. Black, S. R. Furney, H. M. Graf, & A. E. Nolte (Eds.). *Philosophical foundations of health education* (pp.207–225). San Francisco, CA: John Wiley & Sons.

Ballon, D. (2003). *Challenges and choices: Finding mental health services in Ontario*. Toronto: Canadian Association for Mental Health.

Bandura, A. (1997). *Self-efficacy: The exercise of control*. New York, NY: W.H. Freeman.

Bannerman, H. (1889). *The little black sambo story book.* Cutchogue, NY: Buccaneer Books.

Bassett-Gunter, R., Yessis, J., Manske, S., & Gleddie, D. (2015). Healthy school communities in Canada. *Health Education Journal, 75*(2), 235–248.

Birch, D. A. (2000). A cooperative approach to promoting health literacy: The current health issues project. *Journal of School Health, 70*(2), 69–71.

Boak, A., Hamilton, H. A., Adlaf, E. M., Henderson, J. L., Mann, R. E. (2016). *The mental health and well-being of Ontario students, 1991–2015: Detailed research findings (CAMH Research Document Series 43).* Toronto, ON: Centre for Addiction and Mental Health.

Booth, D (1994). *Story drama. Reading, writing, and role playing across the curriculum.* Markham, ON: Pembroke Publishers Ltd.

Brellochs, C. (1995). *Ingredients for success, comprehensive school-based health centers*. New York, NY: School Health Policy Initiative.

Bronfenbrenner, U. (2005). *Making human beings: Biological perspectives on creating human beings.* Thousand Oaks, CA: Sage.

Bronfenbrenner, U., & Morris, P. A. (1998). The ecology of developmental processes. In W. Damon & R. M. Lerner (Eds). *Handbook of child psychology. Vol 1. Theoretical models of human development.* (5th ed., pp.993–1028). New York, NY: John Wiley.

Burgstahler, S. (2015). *Universal design: Process, principles and applications.* University of Washington. Available at: http://www.washington.edu/doit/sites/default/files/atoms/files/Universal_Design%20Process%20Principles%20and%20Applications.pdf

Canadian Association for School Health and Others. (2007). Canadian Consensus Statement on Comprehensive School Health (Revised Edition). Surrey, BC.

Canadian Institute for Health Information (2016). Available at: http://www.cihi.ca/en/health-spending

Centre for Addiction and Mental Health (2012). *Educating students about drug use and mental health—risk and protective factors: youth and substance abuse.* Available at: http://www.camh.ca/en/education/teachers_school_programs/secondary_education/Pages/curriculum_risk-protect.aspx

Collaborative for Academic, Social and Emotional Learning. (2012). *Effective social and emotional learning programs.* Chicago.

Comprehensive School Health. (2008). Public Health Agency of Canada. Available at: http://www.phac-aspc.gc.ca/dca-dea/7-18yrs-ans/comphealth-eng.php (Last modified on September 29, 2008).

Costantini, L. (2013). Parent engagement. *EdCan Network.* Available at: https://www.edcan.ca/articles/parent-engagement/

Deslandes, R. (2006). Designing and implementing school, family, and community collaboration programs in Quebec, Canada. *School Community Journal, 16*(1), 81–106.

Dewey, J. (1995). *Intelligence in human behavior.* Whitefish, MO: Kessinger Publishing.

Dohmen, J. (2003). Philosophers on the "art of living." *Journal of Happiness Studies, 4,* 351–371.

Drummond, D. (2011). Therapy or surgery? A prescription for Canada's health system. Report submitted to the C.D. Howe Institute. Toronto, ON. Available at: https://www.cdhowe.org/pdf/Benefactors_Lecture_2011.pdf

Epstein, J. L. et al. (2002). *School, family, and community partnerships. Your handbook for action.* Thousand Oaks, CA: Sage.

Epstein, J. L., & Salinas, K. C. (2004). Schools as learning communities. *Educational Leadership, 61*(8), 12–18.

Eugenides, J. (2002). *Middlesex.* London, Bloomsbury.

Ferland, A. Y. (2015). Leadership skills are associated with health behaviours among Canadian children. *Health Promotion International,* 1–10.

Ferguson, M. (1980). *The Aquarian conspiracy. Personal and social transformation in the 1980s.* Los Angeles, CA: J. P. Tarcher.

Freire, P. (1983). *Pedagogy in process: The letters to Guinea-Bissau.* New York, NY: Continuum.

Friedland, S. (1999). Violence Reduction? Start with School Culture. *School Administrator, 56*(6), 14–16.

Friere, P., & Macedo, D. (1987). *Literacy: Reading the word and the world.* Westport, CT: Bergin & Garvey.

Fung, C., Kuhle, S., Lu, C., Purcell, M., Schwartz, M., Storey, K. et al. (2012). From "best practice" to "next practice": The effectiveness of school-based health promotion in improving healthy eating and physical activity and preventing childhood obesity. *International Journal of Behavioral Nutrition & Physical Activity*, 9, 27.

Geringer, J. (2003). Reflections on professional development: Toward higher-quality teaching and learning. *Phi Delta Kappan, 84*(5), 373–377.

Gleddie, D. L. (2012). The devil is in the details: Process and policy in the Battle River Project. *Health Education Journal*, *71*(1), 28–36. doi: 10.1177/0017896910383557

Glouberman, S. (2001). *Towards a new perspective on health and health policy.* Report submitted to the Health Network, Canadian Policy Research Networks. Ottawa, ON. Available at: http://rcrpp.org/documents/2686_en.pdf

Goleman, D. (1995). *Emotional intelligence*. New York, NY: Bantam Books.

Golenbock, P. (1990). *Teammates*. Orlando, FL: Harcourt.

Goodall, J. (2006). *Harvest for hope: A guide to mindful eating*. Grand Central Publishing.

Goodall, J. (2008). Tale of the giveaway buffalo. In A. Peck (Ed.), *Bread, body, spirit: Finding the sacred in food* (pp.38-41). Woodstock, TN: SkyLight Paths Publishing.

Gunther, R., Manske, S., Yessis, J., & Gleddie, D. L. (2015). Healthy school communities in Canada. *Health Education Journal, 75*(2), 235–248.

Habermas, J. (1990). *Moral consciousness and communitive action.* Cambridge, UK: Polity Press.

Hart, B., & Risley, T. R. (1995). *Meaningful differences in the everyday experience of young American children*. Baltimore: Paul H. Books.

Henderson, A. T., & Mapp, K. L. (2002). *A new wave of evidence. The impact of school, family, and community connections on student achievement.* National Centre for Family and Community Schools. Available at: https://www.sedl.org/connections/resources/evidence.pdf

Joint Committee on National Health Education Standards. (1995). *Achieving health literacy: An investment in the future*. Atlanta, GA: American Cancer Society.

Joint Consortium for School Health (2009a). *Addressing substance use in Canadian schools. Responding to the needs of higher risk youth.* Joint Consortium for School Health. Available at: https://www.jcsh-cces.ca/upload/JCSH%20Substance%20Use%20Toolkit%20Higher%20Risk%20Youth%20v1.pdf

Joint Consortium for School Health (2009b). *Addressing substance use in Canadian schools. School-family-community partnerships.* Joint Consortium for School Health. Available at: https://www.jcsh-cces.ca/upload/JCSH%20Substance%20Use%20Toolkit%20SchoolFamily-Community%20v1.pdf

Joint Consortium for School Health. (2005). *What is comprehensive school health?* Summerside, PE. Available at: http://www.jcsh-cces.ca/index.php/about/comprehensive-school-health

Joint Consortium for School Health (JCSH). (2008). *What is comprehensive school health?* Available at: http://www.jcsh-cces.ca/upload/JCSH%20CSH%20Framework%20FINAL%20Nov%2008.pdf

King, A., Boyce, W., & King, M. (1999). *Trends in the health of Canadian youth—Summary booklet*. Ottawa: Health Canada.

Kohn, A. (1996). *Beyond discipline: From compliance to community.* Alexandria, VA: Association for Supervision and Curriculum Development.

Lane, R. E. (1994). Quality of life and quality of persons. A new role for government? *Political Theory, 22,* 219–252.

Lee, E. (1994). Taking multicultural anti-racist education seriously: An interview with educator Enid Lee. In B. Bigelow, L. Christensen, S. Karp, B. Milner, & B. Peterson (Eds.), *Rethinking our classrooms* (Vol 1). Milwaukee, WI: Rethinking Schools.

Lerner, R. M., & Benson, P. L. (2003). *Developmental assets and asset-building communities: Implications for research, policy, and practice*. Norwell, MA: Kluwer Academic.

Mandigo, J. (2007). A Tribute to Dr. Andy Anderson November 24, 1950—August 30, 2007. *Physical & Health Education Journal, 73*(3), 45–46.

Mandigo, J. (2002). The MOVEment towards active schools. *Physical and Health Education Journal, 68*(3), 4–10.

Marzano, R. (2004). *Building background knowledge for academic achievement.* Alexandria, VA: Association for Supervision and Curriculum Development.

McCall, D. (1999). Comprehensive school health: Help for teachers from the community. *Physical and Health Education Journal, 65*(1), 4–9.

McCall, D. (2004). *The role of the school in promoting mental health.* Canadian Association for School Health.

McCall, D. & Andrew, C. (2006). Approaches to and research on school health promotion. Joint Consortium for School Health. Summerside, PE. Available at: http://www.jcsh-cces.ca/upload/approaches_research_school_health.pdf.

McDonald, L., & Frey, H. E. (1999). Families and schools together: Building relationships. *Juvenile Justice Bulletin,* November, 1–20.

Ministry of Education. (2004). M*aking meaning. Making a difference*. Aukland, NZ: Ministry of Education. Available at: http://www.tki.org.nz/r/health/cia/make_meaning/index_e.html

Morrison, W., & Peterson, P. (2013). *Schools as a setting for promoting positive mental health. Better practices and perspectives* (2nd ed.). Joint Consortium for School Health. Available at: https://www.jcsh-cces.ca/upload/JCSH%20Best%20Practice_Eng_Jan21.pdf

Murray, N. G., Low, B. J., Hollis, C., Cross, A. W., & Davis, S. M. (2007). Coordinated school health programs and academic achievement: A systematic review of the literature. *Journal of School Health, 77*(9), 589–600.

Musschenga, A. W. (1994). Quality of life and handicapped people. In L. Nordenfelt (Ed.), *Concepts and measurement of quality of life in health care* (pp.181–198). Boston, MA: Kluwer Academic Publishers.

Nadirova, A. B. (2014). *Analysis of provincial achievement test results for the schools participating in APPLE Schools.* Edmonton, AB, Canada: APPLE Schools Foundation.

Nussbaum, M. C. (1990). Aristotelian social democracy. In R. B. Douglass, G. M. Mara, & H. S. Richardson (Eds.). *Liberalism and good* (pp.203–252). New York, NY: Routledge.

Nutbeam, D. (2000). Health literacy as a public health goal: A challenge for contemporary health education and communication strategies in the 21st century. *Health Promotion International, 15*, 259–267.

Ontario Ministry of Education. (2012). *Supporting minds. An educator's guide to promoting students' mental health and well-being.* Toronto, ON: Author. Available from: http://www.edu.gov.on.ca/eng/document/reports/SupportingMinds.pdf

ParticipACTION. (2015). *2015 ParticipACTION report card on physical activity for children and youth.* Toronto, ON: Participaction.

Pérez, J., de Cuéllar, L. A., Fall, Y. K., Furgler, K., Furtado, C., Goulandris, N., Griffin, K., ulHaq, M., Jelin, E., Kamba, A., Magga, O. H., Mikhalkov, N., Nakane, C., & Takla, L. (1997). *Our creative diversity*. New Delhi, India: Oxford & IBH Publishing Co.

Peterson, B. (1994). The challenge of classroom discipline. In B. Bigelow, L. Christensen, S. Karp, B. Miner & B. Peterson (Eds.), *Rethinking our classrooms: Teaching for equity and justice*, (p.34–35). Milwaukee, WI: Rethinking Schools, Ltd.

Postman, N (1996). *The end of education.* New York: Vintage Books.

Public Health Agency of Canada. (2007). Comprehensive school health model. Available at: http://www.phac-aspc.gc.ca/dca-dea/7-18yrs-ans/comphealth-eng.php

Raffan, J. (2000). *Nature nurtures: Investigating the potential for school grounds. Ottawa, ON:* Evergreen. Available at: http://www.evergreen.ca/downloads/pdfs/Nature-Nurtures.pdf

Rawls, J. (1971). *A theory of justice*. Boston: Harvard University Press.

Renwick R., & Brown, I. (1996). The centre for health promotion's conceptual approach to quality of life: being, belonging and becoming. In R. Renwick et al. (Eds.). *Quality of life in health promotion and rehabilitation. Conceptual approaches, issues, and applications.* Thousand Oaks, CA: Sage Publications.

Ritchart, R. (2002). *Intellectual character: What it is, why it matters, and how to get it.* San Francisco, CA: Jossey-Bass.

Roberts, E. M. (2015). Implementing comprehensive school health in Alberta, Canada: The principal's role. *Health Promotion International*, 1–10 .

Salas, L. M. (1997). Violence and aggression in the schools of Colombia, El Salvador, Guatemala, Nicaragua, and Peru. In T. Ohsako (Ed.). *Violence at school: Global issues and interventions* (pp.110–127). Lausanne: UNESCO.

Samdal, O., Nutbeam, D., Wold, B., & Kansas, L. (1998). Achieving health and educational goals through schools—a study of the importance of the school climate and the students' satisfaction with school. *Health Education Research, 13*, 383–398.

Sanders, M. G. (2001). A study of the role of "community" in comprehensive school, family, and community partnership programs. *The Elementary School Journal, 102*, 19–34.

Sanders, M. G., & Harvey, A. (2002). Beyond the school walls: A case study of principal leadership for school-community collaboration. *Teachers College Record, 104*(7), 1345–1368.

Schwartz, M. K. (2010). *Tailoring and implementing comprehensive school health: The Alberta project promoting active living and healthy eating in schools. 2*, 1–9.

Seligman, M. (1998). *Learned optimism. How to change your mind and your life.* New York, NY: Random House.

Sheldon, S. B. (2003). Linking school family community partnership in urban elementary schools to student achievement on state tests. *The Urban Review, 35*, 149–165.

Sheppard, J. & Wray, A. (2012). Champions for health promoting schools. *Physical and Health Education Journal,* 78(2).

Simon, R. (1992). *Teaching against the grain: Texts for a pedagogy of possibility*. New York, NY: Bergin & Garvey.

Spitters, H. S. (2009). Parents' and students' support for policies that promote healthy eating and active living. *Physical and Health Education Journal*, 30–34.

Stephens, T., & Graham, D. F. (1993). *Canada's health promotion survey: Technical report.* Ottawa, ON: Minister of Supply and Services.

Storey, K. M., Montemurro, G., & Schwartz, M. (2015). Preparing school health facilitators: Building competence and confidence for a new role. *7*.

Storey, K. S. (2011). Teachers' perceptions of the Alberta project promoting active living and healthy eating: APPLE schools. *Health and Education Academic Journal, 3*, 1–18.

Suhrcke, M, & Nieves, C. (2011). *The impact of health and health behaviours on educational outcomes in high-income countries: A review of the evidence.* Copenhagen: WHO Regional Office for Europe.

Symons, C., Cincelli, B., James, T. C, Groff, P. (1997). Bridging student health risks and academic achievement through comprehensive school health programs. *Journal of School Health, 67*, 220–227.

Sze, S. (1998). WHO: From small beginnings. *World Health Forum, 9*, 29–34.

Tasker, G. (2000). *Social and ethical issues in sexuality education: A resource for health education teachers of year 12 and 13 students.* Christchurch: Christchurch College of Education.

Tran, B. O. (2014). Life course impact of school-based promotion of healthy eating and active living to prevent childhood obesity. *Health Promotion International.*

Toulouse, P. R. (2016). *What matters in Indigenous education? Implementing a vision committed to holism, diversity and engagement.* Toronto, ON: People for Education.

United Nations (2015). *The millenium development goals report.* Geneva, Switzerland.

UNICEF (2012). *Global evaluation of life skills.* Retrieved September 22, 2015 from United Nations Website: http://www.unicef.org/evaluation/files/USA-2012-011-1_GLSEE.pdf

Vander Ploeg, K. M., Maximova, K., McGavock, J., Davis, W., & Veuglers, P. (2014). Do school-based physical activity inteventions increase or reduce inequalities in health? *Social Science and Medicine, 112*, 80–87 .

Vander Ploeg, K. W., McGavock, J., Maximova, K., & Veugelers, P. S. (2014). School-based health promotion and physical activity during and after school hours. *Pediatrics, 133,* e371–e378.

Veenhoven, R. (2000). The four qualities of life: Ordering concepts and measures of the good life. *Journal of Happiness Studies, 1*, 1–39.

Veugelers, P. (2014). *REAL Kids Alberta.* Retreived August 2015 from website: www.realkidsalberta.ca. August 2015.

Veugelers, P. F., & Fitzgerald, A. L. (2005). Effectiveness of school programs in preventing childhood obesity: A multilevel comparison. *American Journal of Public Health*, 432–437.

Veugelers, P. S., Schwartz, M. (2010). Comprehensive school health in Canada. *Canadian Journal of Public Health, 101, Supplement 2*, S4–S8.

Wharf Higgins, J., Gaul, C., Gibbons, S., & Van Gyn, G. (2003). Factors influencing physical activity levels among Canadian youth. *Canadian Journal of Public Health, 94*, 45–51.

Wilkinson, S. (1996). *Feminist social psychologies: International perspectives.* Buckingham, UK: Open University Press.

World Health Organization. (1997). *The Health Promoting School—An investment in education, health and democracy*. Conference Report (Greece, May 1–5). Copenhagen, Denmark: WHO Regional Office for Europe.

World Health Organization. (1998). *Health-promoting schools—A healthy setting for living, learning and working.* Geneva, Switzerland: World Health Organization Division of Health Promotion, Education and Communication. Available at http://www.who.int/school_youth_health/media/en/92.pdf

World Health Organization (2003). *Skills for health: Skills-based health education including life skills: An important component of a child-friendly/health-promoting school.* The World Health Organization's Information Series on School Health, Document 9.

World Health Organization (1986). *Ottawa charter for health promotion*. First International Conference on Health Promotion, Session 21 November. (Report No. WHO/HPR/HEP/95.1) Available at http://www.who.int/hpr/NPH/docs/ottawa_charter_hp.pdf

World Health Organization. (2000). *Promoting active living in and through schools: Policy statement and guidelines for action.* Report of a WHO Meeting, Session May 25–27, 1998, Esbjerg, Denmark. (Report No. WHO/NMH/NPH/00.4) Available at http://www.hpclearinghouse.ca/downloads/WHO_Promoting_active_living_in_schools.pdf

World Health Organization. (1986). *The Ottawa charter for health promotion.* Report of a WHO International Conference on Health Promotion, November 21, 1986, Ottawa, ON. Available at http://www.who.int/healthpromotion/conferences/previous/ottawa/en/

Wright, J. (2006). Physical education research from postmodern, post structural and postcolonial perspectives. In D. Kirk, D. Macdonald, & M. O'Sullivan (Eds). *The handbook of physical education* (pp.59–75). London, UK: Sage.

Index

P

Q

R

S